OWEN HUNTER

Keratosis Pilaris

Your Comprehensive Blueprint for Diagnosis and Treatment

Contents

INTRODUCTION

Keratosis Pilaris: A Journey to Smoother, Healthier Skin

Welcome to the world of Keratosis Pilaris (KP), a common skin condition that affects millions of people worldwide. If you or someone you know has been struggling with rough, bumpy skin that resembles goosebumps or chicken skin, you've come to the right place. This book is designed to be your comprehensive guide to understanding, managing, and ultimately thriving with Keratosis Pilaris.

Keratosis Pilaris is a harmless but often frustrating skin condition that occurs when dead skin cells and keratin build up in the hair follicles, causing small, rough bumps to appear on the skin's surface. These bumps commonly appear on the upper arms, thighs, cheeks, and buttocks, and can be accompanied by redness, dryness, and itching. While Keratosis Pilaris is not physically harmful, it can take a toll on one's self-esteem and confidence, leading to feelings of self-consciousness and even social anxiety.

Despite its prevalence, Keratosis Pilaris remains a relatively misunderstood condition. Many people with KP feel alone in their struggles, not realizing that they are part of a large community of individuals who share the same challenges. This lack of awareness can make it difficult for those with KP to find reliable information, effective treatments, and the emotional support they need to manage their condition.

That's where this book comes in. Our goal is to provide you with a comprehensive, up-to-date, and compassionate guide to navigating life with Keratosis Pilaris. Whether you've been recently diagnosed, have been living with KP for years, or are supporting a loved one with the condition, this book is designed to empower you with the knowledge, tools, and strategies you need to take control of your skin health and live your best life.

Throughout these pages, we'll dive deep into the science behind Keratosis Pilaris, exploring its causes, symptoms, and the various factors that can contribute to its development. We'll provide you with a clear understanding of what's happening beneath the surface of your skin, and why KP manifests the way it does.

But we won't stop there. We understand that living with Keratosis Pilaris is about more than just the physical symptoms. It's about the emotional impact of having a visible skin condition, the frustration of trying countless treatments without success, and the daily challenges of maintaining a consistent skincare routine. That's why we've dedicated entire chapters to the psychological aspects of living with KP, offering coping strategies, self-care tips, and resources for finding support and building a positive body image.

One of the most significant challenges faced by those with Keratosis Pilaris is finding effective treatments. With so many products and remedies marketed toward KP, it can be overwhelming to know where to start. In this book, we'll cut through the noise and provide you with a comprehensive overview of the most proven treatments for Keratosis Pilaris, from gentle skincare routines and over-the-counter products to professional procedures and natural remedies. We'll help you understand the pros and cons of each approach, and guide you in developing a personalized treatment plan that works for your unique skin type and lifestyle.

But effective treatment is only one piece of the puzzle. To truly manage Keratosis Pilaris, it's essential to address the broader factors that influence skin health, such as diet, hydration, and lifestyle habits. We'll explore the role of nutrition in managing KP, offering practical tips for incorporating skin-friendly foods into your diet and identifying potential trigger foods to avoid. We'll also discuss the importance of staying hydrated, managing stress, and maintaining a balanced lifestyle to support overall skin health.

Throughout the book, we'll be sharing real-life stories and testimonials from individuals living with Keratosis Pilaris. These stories serve as a powerful reminder that you are not alone in your journey, and that it is possible to achieve smoother, healthier skin and a more positive self-image. We hope that by reading these stories, you'll feel inspired, empowered, and connected to a community of people who understand what you're going through.

As we look to the future, we'll explore the latest research and innovations in Keratosis Pilaris treatment, offering a glimpse into the promising new therapies and technologies on the horizon. We'll also discuss the importance of advocating for greater awareness and research funding for KP, and provide resources for getting involved in the fight for better treatments and support.

Whether you're reading this book from cover to cover or using it as a reference guide to dip into as needed, our aim is to provide you with the most comprehensive, accurate, and empowering information available on Keratosis Pilaris. We hope that by arming you with knowledge, strategies, and support, we can help you take control of your skin health, boost your confidence, and live your best life.

So, let's dive in and begin your journey to smoother, healthier skin. Remember, you are not alone, and with the right tools and mindset, you have the power to manage Keratosis Pilaris and thrive. Let's get started!

CHAPTER 1

Understanding Keratosis Pilaris: What It Is and Why It Occurs

1.1 Defining Keratosis Pilaris

Keratosis Pilaris (KP) is a common skin condition that affects an estimated 40-50% of the adult population and up to 80% of adolescents. It is characterized by the appearance of small, rough, bumpy patches of skin, often described as resembling goosebumps or chicken skin. These bumps, known as papules, are typically skin-colored or red and appear most commonly on the upper arms, thighs, cheeks, and buttocks.

Despite its prevalence, Keratosis Pilaris remains a relatively misunderstood condition, with many people unaware that their bumpy skin has a name or that effective treatments are available. This lack of awareness can lead to feelings of self-consciousness, frustration, and even embarrassment for those living with KP.

At its core, Keratosis Pilaris is a disorder of keratinization, the process by which the skin produces and sheds keratin, a tough, protective protein that makes up the outer layer of skin. In people with KP, this process goes awry, leading to the buildup of keratin and dead skin cells in the hair follicles, which ultimately results in the formation of the characteristic bumps.

It's important to note that Keratosis Pilaris is a benign condition, meaning it is not harmful to your overall health. It is not contagious, and it does not indicate poor hygiene or an underlying disease. However, the appearance of KP can be aesthetically bothersome and can lead to significant emotional distress for some individuals.

1.2 Causes and Risk Factors

To effectively manage Keratosis Pilaris, it's essential to understand the underlying causes and risk factors that contribute to its development. While the exact cause of KP remains unknown, researchers have identified several key factors that play a role in its onset and severity.

One of the primary factors believed to contribute to Keratosis Pilaris is genetics. Studies have shown that KP tends to run in families, suggesting that there may be an inherited component to the condition. If you have a parent or sibling with Keratosis Pilaris, you may be more likely to develop it yourself.

In addition to genetics, hormonal changes are thought to play a significant role in the development and exacerbation of Keratosis Pilaris. Many people with KP report that their symptoms worsen during puberty, pregnancy, and menopause, times when the body undergoes significant hormonal shifts. This connection suggests that hormones like androgens and estrogens may influence the skin's keratin production and shedding processes.

Environmental factors can also contribute to the severity of Keratosis Pilaris. Cold, dry weather and low humidity levels can exacerbate KP by dehydrating the skin, making it more prone to keratin buildup and irritation. On the other hand, hot, humid weather can sometimes improve KP symptoms by keeping the skin moist and facilitating the shedding of dead skin cells.

Certain skin care practices and products may also aggravate Keratosis

Pilaris. Harsh soaps, exfoliants, and scrubs can strip the skin of its natural oils, disrupting its protective barrier and leading to further dryness and irritation. Similarly, products containing alcohol, fragrances, and other potential irritants can worsen KP symptoms in some individuals.

It's worth noting that while these factors can influence the development and severity of Keratosis Pilaris, not everyone with these risk factors will develop the condition. Conversely, some people may develop KP without any identifiable risk factors. The complex interplay between genetics, hormones, environment, and individual skin characteristics makes Keratosis Pilaris a highly variable condition that manifests differently from person to person.

Understanding the potential causes and risk factors for Keratosis Pilaris is an essential first step in developing an effective management plan. By identifying your own unique triggers and risk factors, you can take proactive steps to minimize flare-ups, optimize your skin care routine, and maintain the overall health and appearance of your skin.

1.3 Symptoms and Variations

Keratosis Pilaris is characterized by a distinct set of symptoms that can vary in severity and appearance from person to person. The hallmark of KP is the presence of small, rough, bumpy patches of skin, typically described as having a sandpaper-like texture. These bumps, known as papules, are usually skin-colored or red and tend to appear in clusters on the upper arms, thighs, cheeks, and buttocks.

Upon closer examination, you may notice that each individual bump is centered around a hair follicle. In fact, Keratosis Pilaris is often referred to as "follicular keratosis" due to its close association with the hair follicles. The bumps may be more pronounced and visible when the skin is dry, and they can sometimes be accompanied by mild itching or a feeling of roughness.

In some cases, the papules of Keratosis Pilaris may take on a more inflamed, reddened appearance. This variation, known as Keratosis Pilaris Rubra, is characterized by red, irritated bumps that may be more tender or itchy than the standard skin-colored papules. Keratosis Pilaris Rubra is more common in individuals with fair, sensitive skin and can be exacerbated by friction from clothing, harsh skin care products, or environmental factors like cold, dry weather.

Another variation of Keratosis Pilaris is known as Keratosis Pilaris Alba. In this subtype, the papules are typically skin-colored or slightly lighter than the surrounding skin, giving the affected areas a more subtle, goosebump-like appearance. Keratosis Pilaris Alba is more common in individuals with darker skin tones and may be less noticeable than the reddened papules of Keratosis Pilaris Rubra.

It's important to note that the severity of Keratosis Pilaris can vary significantly from person to person and can even fluctuate over time within the same individual. Some people may experience mild, barely noticeable bumps, while others may have more extensive, visibly rough patches of skin. The severity of KP can be influenced by a variety of factors, including genetics, hormonal changes, environmental conditions, and skin care practices.

In addition to the physical symptoms of Keratosis Pilaris, many people with the condition also experience emotional symptoms like self-consciousness, embarrassment, and frustration. The appearance of rough, bumpy skin can lead to feelings of insecurity and a reluctance to expose affected areas, particularly during warmer months when shorts and sleeveless tops are more common. These emotional symptoms can be just as challenging to manage as the physical ones and underscore the importance of developing a comprehensive approach to KP management that addresses both the skin and the mind.

If you suspect that you may have Keratosis Pilaris, it's essential to familiarize yourself with the typical symptoms and variations of the condition. By understanding what to look for and how KP can manifest, you'll be better equipped to identify your own unique symptoms, track changes over time, and develop an effective management plan in collaboration with your dermatologist or skincare professional.

Remember, while the symptoms of Keratosis Pilaris can be bothersome and frustrating, they are ultimately harmless and do not pose a threat to your overall health. With the right combination of self-care, professional guidance, and emotional support, it is possible to manage KP effectively and maintain healthy, comfortable skin. In the following chapters, we'll delve deeper into the various strategies and treatments available for managing Keratosis Pilaris, empowering you with the knowledge and tools you need to take control of your skin health and live your best life.

CHAPTER 2

Diagnosing Keratosis Pilaris: When to Seek Medical Advice

2.1 Self-Diagnosis vs. Professional Diagnosis

If you've been experiencing rough, bumpy patches of skin on your upper arms, thighs, cheeks, or buttocks, you may be wondering if you have Keratosis Pilaris (KP). While it can be tempting to self-diagnose based on the appearance of your skin and the information you've gathered from various sources, it's essential to understand the limitations and potential risks of self-diagnosis.

Keratosis Pilaris is a relatively common and benign skin condition, and in many cases, it can be accurately identified based on its distinctive appearance and texture. However, there are several other skin conditions that can mimic the symptoms of KP, making self-diagnosis a tricky proposition.

Some conditions that may resemble Keratosis Pilaris include:

1. Folliculitis: This is an inflammation of the hair follicles caused by bacterial or fungal infection. It can result in small, red, sometimes itchy or painful bumps around the hair follicles.

2. Eczema: Also known as atopic dermatitis, eczema is a chronic skin condition characterized by dry, itchy, and inflamed skin. In some cases,

eczema can cause rough, bumpy patches that may resemble KP.

3. Psoriasis: Psoriasis is an autoimmune condition that causes the rapid buildup of skin cells, leading to the formation of scaly, itchy, and sometimes painful patches. While psoriasis typically appears in larger, more inflamed patches than KP, it can sometimes be mistaken for severe Keratosis Pilaris.

4. Acne: While acne is most commonly associated with the face, it can also appear on the body, particularly in areas like the upper arms and back. The bumps and pustules of body acne can sometimes be confused with the papules of Keratosis Pilaris.

5. Keratosis Pilaris Atrophicans: This is a rare variant of KP that causes more pronounced, inflammatory papules that may lead to scarring and skin atrophy (thinning). It is often more resistant to standard KP treatments and may require more aggressive medical intervention.

Given the potential for misdiagnosis, it's always advisable to seek professional input from a dermatologist or other qualified skincare professional if you suspect you may have Keratosis Pilaris. A trained professional can perform a thorough examination of your skin, taking into account factors like the appearance, texture, and distribution of the bumps, as well as your medical history and any other relevant symptoms.

In most cases, a dermatologist can diagnose Keratosis Pilaris based on a simple visual examination. However, in rare instances where the diagnosis is uncertain, or there is suspicion of an underlying condition, your dermatologist may recommend additional tests, such as a skin biopsy, to rule out other possibilities and confirm the diagnosis.

Seeking professional diagnosis not only ensures that you receive an accurate assessment of your skin condition but also opens the door to personalized treatment recommendations and ongoing support from a knowledgeable skincare provider. Your dermatologist can help you navigate the various treatment options available for Keratosis Pilaris, taking into account factors like the severity of your symptoms, your skin type, and your individual preferences and lifestyle.

2.2 Differential Diagnosis: Ruling Out Similar Skin Conditions

As mentioned earlier, several skin conditions can mimic the appearance of Keratosis Pilaris, making differential diagnosis an essential step in the evaluation process. Differential diagnosis involves systematically considering and ruling out other possible conditions based on their unique characteristics and the patient's overall clinical picture.

When differentiating Keratosis Pilaris from other similar skin conditions, dermatologists will typically consider the following factors:

1. Location: Keratosis Pilaris most commonly appears on the upper arms, thighs, cheeks, and buttocks. While other conditions like folliculitis and acne can also affect these areas, they may have a more widespread distribution or appear in other locations not typically associated with KP.

2. Appearance: The papules of Keratosis Pilaris are typically small (less than 1mm in diameter), uniform in size and shape, and centered around hair follicles. They may be skin-colored, red, or slightly hyperpigmented, depending on the individual's skin tone and the severity of the condition. In contrast, conditions like folliculitis may present with larger, more inflamed, or pustular bumps, while eczema and psoriasis often cause larger patches of dry, scaly, or inflamed skin.

3. Texture: Keratosis Pilaris is characterized by a distinct rough, sandpaper-like texture, which is caused by the buildup of keratin in the hair follicles. Other conditions may cause different textures, such as the grittiness of acne or the smoothness of eczema patches.

4. Symptoms: While Keratosis Pilaris can sometimes cause mild itching or dryness, it is typically asymptomatic. In contrast, conditions like folliculitis, eczema, and psoriasis often cause more significant itching, burning, or discomfort.

5. Response to treatment: Keratosis Pilaris typically responds well to gentle exfoliation, moisturization, and the use of keratolytic agents like alpha-hydroxy acids (AHAs) or urea. If a patient's skin condition does not improve with standard KP treatments, it may suggest an alternative diagnosis that requires a different approach.

By carefully evaluating these factors and considering the patient's overall medical history and any additional symptoms, dermatologists can effectively rule out other conditions and arrive at an accurate diagnosis of Keratosis Pilaris.

It's worth noting that in some cases, Keratosis Pilaris may coexist with other skin conditions like atopic dermatitis or ichthyosis vulgaris. In these situations, a comprehensive treatment plan that addresses both conditions may be necessary to achieve optimal results.

If you're unsure about your diagnosis or have concerns about your skin condition, don't hesitate to seek professional advice. A dermatologist can provide you with a definitive diagnosis, rule out other possibilities, and develop a personalized treatment plan to help you manage your symptoms and improve the overall health and appearance of your skin.

2.3 What to Expect During a Dermatologist Visit

If you've decided to seek professional evaluation for your suspected Keratosis Pilaris, you may be wondering what to expect during your dermatologist visit. While the specific details of your appointment may vary depending on your individual situation and the practices of your chosen provider, there are some general elements that are common to most dermatological evaluations for KP.

When you arrive for your appointment, you'll typically be asked to fill out some paperwork, including a medical history form and any necessary insurance or payment information. This is a good opportunity to gather your thoughts and make note of any specific concerns or questions you'd like to discuss with your dermatologist.

Once you're called back to the examination room, your dermatologist will likely begin by asking you a series of questions about your skin concerns, your medical history, and any treatments you've tried in the past. They may ask about the onset and duration of your symptoms, any factors that seem to improve or worsen your condition, and any other health issues or medications that could be relevant to your skin health.

Next, your dermatologist will perform a thorough visual examination of your skin, focusing on the areas where you've noticed the rough, bumpy patches characteristic of Keratosis Pilaris. They may use a magnifying lens or specialized lighting to get a closer look at the texture and distribution of the papules, as well as any other notable features of your skin.

In most cases, this visual examination will be sufficient for your dermatologist to diagnose Keratosis Pilaris and differentiate it from other similar conditions. However, if there is any uncertainty or concern about the possibility of an underlying condition, your dermatologist may recommend additional tests, such as a skin biopsy, to confirm the diagnosis and rule out other possibilities.

Once a definitive diagnosis has been made, your dermatologist will discuss treatment options with you. They may recommend a combination of self-care measures, such as gentle exfoliation and moisturization, as well as topical medications or in-office treatments designed to improve the texture and appearance of your skin.

Your dermatologist should take the time to explain each treatment option in detail, including its potential benefits, risks, and side effects, as well as any necessary precautions or follow-up care. They should also provide you with personalized guidance on how to incorporate these treatments into your daily skincare routine and what kind of results you can expect over time.

Throughout the appointment, don't hesitate to ask questions or voice any concerns you may have about your diagnosis, treatment options, or overall skin health. A good dermatologist will be happy to provide you with the information and support you need to feel confident and empowered in managing your Keratosis Pilaris.

At the end of your visit, your dermatologist may schedule a follow-up appointment to monitor your progress and make any necessary adjustments to your treatment plan. They may also provide you with educational resources, product recommendations, or referrals to other specialists if needed.

Remember, seeking professional evaluation for your Keratosis Pilaris is an important step in taking control of your skin health and finding the solutions that work best for you. With the right diagnosis, personalized treatment plan, and ongoing support from your dermatologist, you can effectively manage your KP symptoms and enjoy the smooth, healthy skin you deserve.

CHAPTER 3

The Emotional Impact of Keratosis Pilaris: Coping Strategies and Support

3.1 Understanding the Psychological Effects

While Keratosis Pilaris (KP) is a physical skin condition, its impact extends far beyond the surface of the skin. For many people living with KP, the emotional and psychological effects can be just as challenging, if not more so, than the physical symptoms themselves.

The visible nature of Keratosis Pilaris can lead to feelings of self-consciousness, embarrassment, and even shame. In a society that often equates clear, smooth skin with beauty and desirability, the presence of rough, bumpy patches can be a significant source of insecurity and low self-esteem.

Many people with KP report feeling anxious or reluctant to expose their affected skin, particularly in social situations or intimate settings. They may avoid wearing short sleeves, shorts, or swimsuits, even in warm weather, for fear of drawing attention to their skin. This self-imposed concealment can lead to feelings of isolation, as well as missed opportunities for social connection and physical activity.

The emotional impact of Keratosis Pilaris can be particularly pronounced during adolescence and young adulthood, when the desire to fit in and conform to societal beauty standards is often at its peak. Teenagers with KP may face teasing, bullying, or unwanted questions about their skin, which can further erode their self-confidence and contribute to feelings of anxiety or depression.

Even in adulthood, the persistence of KP can be a source of frustration and disappointment. Many people with KP report feeling like they've tried every treatment available without success, leading to a sense of hopelessness or resignation. The chronic nature of the condition can also be emotionally taxing, as the constant need for management and concealment can feel like an endless burden.

It's essential to recognize that these emotional responses to Keratosis Pilaris are valid and understandable. In a culture that places so much emphasis on physical appearance, it's natural to feel self-conscious or anxious about a visible skin condition. However, it's equally important to remember that KP does not define your worth or value as a person, and that there are strategies and resources available to help you cope with the emotional impact of the condition.

One of the first steps in managing the psychological effects of Keratosis Pilaris is to acknowledge and validate your feelings. Give yourself permission to feel frustrated, anxious, or self-conscious at times, without judgment or self-blame. Recognize that these emotions are a normal response to a challenging situation, and that they do not reflect any weakness or inadequacy on your part.

It can also be helpful to reframe your perspective on Keratosis Pilaris and its impact on your life. While it's natural to focus on the negative aspects of the condition, try to also acknowledge the ways in which it may have strengthened your resilience, empathy, or appreciation for inner beauty. Many people with KP find that their experiences with the condition have made them more compassionate and accepting of others' differences and struggles.

Finally, don't hesitate to seek support and guidance from others who understand what you're going through. Whether it's through online forums, support groups, or individual therapy, connecting with others who share your experiences can be a powerful source of validation, encouragement, and practical advice.

Remember, the emotional impact of Keratosis Pilaris is just as real and significant as the physical symptoms, and deserves the same level of attention and care. By acknowledging your feelings, reframing your perspective, and seeking support when needed, you can develop the resilience and self-compassion necessary to thrive in spite of KP.

3.2 Building Self-Confidence and Body Positivity

One of the most important aspects of managing the emotional impact of Keratosis Pilaris is learning to cultivate self-confidence and body positivity. This involves shifting your focus from the perceived flaws or imperfections of your skin to a more holistic and accepting view of yourself as a whole person.

Building self-confidence with KP starts with challenging the negative beliefs and assumptions you may hold about your skin and appearance. Many people with KP have internalized messages from society, media, or even well-meaning family members that suggest that their skin is unattractive, abnormal, or something to be ashamed of. These messages can be deeply ingrained and difficult to overcome, but it's essential to recognize that they are based on narrow and unrealistic standards of beauty, rather than on your inherent worth as a person.

One way to start challenging these negative beliefs is to practice self-compassion. This means treating yourself with the same kindness, understanding, and forgiveness that you would extend to a good friend or loved one. When you notice yourself engaging in negative self-talk or self-criticism about your skin, try to reframe those thoughts in a more compassionate and understanding way.

For example, instead of thinking "My skin is so ugly and embarrassing," try reframing the thought as "My skin is just one part of who I am, and it doesn't define my worth or value as a person." Or, instead of "I'll never have perfect skin," try "My skin is unique and beautiful in its own way, even with KP."

Another important aspect of building self-confidence with Keratosis Pilaris is learning to focus on the aspects of yourself and your life that bring you joy, fulfillment, and a sense of purpose. This might include your talents, passions, relationships, or personal achievements. By shifting your focus to these positive aspects of your identity, you can start to develop a more balanced and accepting view of yourself that isn't solely defined by your skin.

It can also be helpful to surround yourself with positive and supportive influences, whether that's friends and family members who appreciate you for who you are, or media and social media accounts that promote diverse and inclusive standards of beauty. Seek out images, stories, and role models that celebrate a wide range of skin types, textures, and appearances, and that emphasize the importance of inner beauty, character, and resilience.

Finally, don't be afraid to take steps to care for and appreciate your skin, even with Keratosis Pilaris. While it's important not to base your entire self-worth on the appearance of your skin, engaging in a gentle and nourishing skincare routine can be a powerful act of self-love and self-care. By taking the time to moisturize, exfoliate, and protect your skin, you're sending yourself the message that your skin is valuable and deserving of care and attention, regardless of its texture or appearance.

Remember, building self-confidence and body positivity with Keratosis

Pilaris is a journey, and it may take time and practice to shift your mindset and beliefs. Be patient and compassionate with yourself, and don't hesitate to seek support and guidance from others who understand what you're going through. With persistence and self-love, it is possible to cultivate a deep and unshakable sense of self-worth, even in the face of KP.

3.3 Finding Support: Online Communities and Resources

One of the most powerful ways to cope with the emotional impact of Keratosis Pilaris is to connect with others who share your experiences and struggles. While KP can feel isolating and lonely at times, it's important to remember that you are not alone, and that there is a vibrant and supportive community of individuals living with this condition.

Online forums and social media groups can be an invaluable resource for people with Keratosis Pilaris, offering a safe and welcoming space to share experiences, ask questions, and offer support and encouragement to others. These communities can be especially helpful for those who may not have access to in-person support groups or who feel uncomfortable discussing their skin concerns with friends or family members.

Some popular online communities for people with Keratosis Pilaris include:

1. Reddit's r/KeratosisPilaris subreddit: This active and engaging community offers a mix of personal stories, treatment advice, and emotional support for people living with KP.

2. Facebook groups: There are numerous Facebook groups dedicated to Keratosis Pilaris, including "Keratosis Pilaris Support Group" and "Keratosis Pilaris Awareness & Support." These groups offer a platform for members to share photos, ask for product recommendations, and connect with others who understand their struggles.

3. Instagram accounts: Many individuals with KP have turned to Instagram to share their experiences and offer support and encouragement to others. Accounts like @keratosispilaris.support and @kp_community offer a mix of personal stories, skincare tips, and body-positive messaging.

In addition to these online communities, there are also numerous websites and resources dedicated to providing information and support for people with Keratosis Pilaris. Some notable examples include:

1. The National Keratosis Pilaris Association (NKPA): This non-profit organization offers a wealth of information on KP, including treatment options, skincare advice, and emotional support resources.

2. The American Academy of Dermatology (AAD): The AAD website offers a comprehensive overview of Keratosis Pilaris, including its causes, symptoms, and treatment options, as well as a directory of board-certified dermatologists.

3. The Mighty: This digital health community offers a platform for people living with a wide range of chronic conditions, including Keratosis Pilaris, to share their stories and connect with others who understand their experiences.

When engaging with online communities and resources, it's important to remember that everyone's experience with Keratosis Pilaris is unique, and what works for one person may not work for another. Be cautious of any advice or recommendations that seem too good to be true, and always consult with a qualified healthcare professional before starting any new treatment or skincare regimen.

It's also important to be mindful of your own emotional boundaries when engaging with online communities. While these spaces can be a valuable source of support and connection, they can also be triggering or overwhelming at times. Don't hesitate to take breaks or step away if you find yourself feeling anxious, stressed, or emotionally drained.

Ultimately, finding support and connection is an essential part of managing the emotional impact of Keratosis Pilaris. Whether it's through online communities, in-person support groups, or individual therapy, having a network of people who understand and validate your experiences can be a powerful source of comfort, encouragement, and resilience. Remember, you are not alone in this journey, and there is always hope and support available, no matter how challenging things may feel in the moment.

CHAPTER 4

Skin Care Routines for Keratosis Pilaris: Cleansing, Exfoliating, and Moisturizing

4.1 Gentle Cleansing Techniques and Products

Establishing a gentle and effective cleansing routine is the foundation of any successful skincare regimen for Keratosis Pilaris (KP). While it may be tempting to scrub or harshly exfoliate the skin in an attempt to remove the rough, bumpy texture, this approach can actually worsen KP symptoms and lead to irritation, redness, and inflammation.

Instead, the key to cleansing skin with Keratosis Pilaris is to use gentle, non-abrasive techniques and products that help to soften and moisturize the skin while removing dirt, oil, and dead skin cells. This approach helps to support the skin's natural barrier function, which is essential for maintaining healthy, resilient skin.

When selecting a cleanser for KP-prone skin, look for products that are:

1. Fragrance-free: Artificial fragrances can be irritating to sensitive skin and may exacerbate KP symptoms. Opt for products that are labeled as "fragrance-free" or "unscented" to minimize the risk of irritation.

2. Sulfate-free: Sulfates, such as sodium lauryl sulfate (SLS) and sodium

laureth sulfate (SLES), are harsh detergents that can strip the skin of its natural oils and disrupt the skin's barrier function. Look for cleansers that are sulfate-free or that contain gentle, non-foaming surfactants like cocamidopropyl betaine or decyl glucoside.

3. pH-balanced: The skin's natural pH is slightly acidic, typically ranging from 4.5 to 6.5. Using cleansers that are too alkaline can disrupt the skin's acid mantle and lead to dryness, irritation, and worsening of KP symptoms. Look for cleansers that are formulated with a pH that is compatible with the skin's natural acidity.

4. Hydrating: Cleansers that contain hydrating ingredients like glycerin, hyaluronic acid, or ceramides can help to moisturize and support the skin's barrier function, which is especially important for those with KP.

Some gentle cleanser options that may be suitable for those with Keratosis Pilaris include:

- Cerave Hydrating Cleanser
    - Vanicream Gentle Facial Cleanser
    - La Roche-Posay Toleriane Hydrating Gentle Cleanser
    - Cetaphil Gentle Skin Cleanser
    - Paula's Choice RESIST Optimal Results Hydrating Cleanser

When cleansing skin with Keratosis Pilaris, it's important to use lukewarm water and gentle, circular motions to avoid excessive friction or irritation. Avoid using harsh scrubs, loofahs, or exfoliating brushes, which can be too abrasive for KP-prone skin. Instead, use your fingertips or a soft washcloth to gently massage the cleanser into the skin, then rinse thoroughly with lukewarm water.

After cleansing, be sure to pat the skin dry with a clean, soft towel, rather than rubbing or scrubbing the skin, which can cause further irritation. If your skin feels tight, dry, or irritated after cleansing, it may be a sign that your cleanser is too harsh or that you're using too much pressure when washing your face. In this case, consider switching to a gentler product or adjusting your cleansing technique.

By incorporating a gentle, hydrating cleanser and using non-abrasive cleansing techniques, you can help to support the health and resilience of your skin, while minimizing the likelihood of worsening KP symptoms. Remember, the goal of cleansing is to remove dirt, oil, and impurities while maintaining the skin's natural moisture balance and barrier function, not to strip or scrub away the bumpy texture of KP.

4.2 Effective Exfoliation Methods

Exfoliation is a crucial step in managing Keratosis Pilaris, as it helps to remove the buildup of keratin and dead skin cells that contribute to the rough, bumpy texture of KP. However, it's important to approach exfoliation with caution, as overly aggressive or frequent exfoliation can actually worsen KP symptoms and lead to irritation, redness, and inflammation.

When it comes to exfoliating skin with Keratosis Pilaris, the key is to use gentle, non-abrasive methods that help to soften and smooth the skin without causing undue irritation. There are two main types of exfoliation: physical exfoliation and chemical exfoliation.

Physical exfoliation involves using a tool or scrub to manually remove dead skin cells from the surface of the skin. While physical exfoliation can be effective for some people with KP, it's important to choose gentle, non-abrasive products and to use them sparingly to avoid over-exfoliating the skin.

Some gentle physical exfoliation options for KP include:

1. Soft washcloths or cleansing cloths: Using a soft, microfiber washcloth or cleansing cloth can provide gentle physical exfoliation without being too abrasive for KP-prone skin. Simply massage the skin gently with the cloth in circular motions, then rinse thoroughly with lukewarm water.

2. Konjac sponges: Made from the root of the konjac plant, these soft, squishy sponges provide gentle exfoliation and can be especially useful for hard-to-reach areas like the upper arms and thighs.

3. Gentle scrubs: If you prefer to use a scrub, look for products that contain gentle, non-abrasive exfoliants like jojoba beads, rice powder, or oatmeal. Avoid scrubs with harsh, jagged particles like walnut shells or apricot kernels, which can be too abrasive for KP-prone skin.

Chemical exfoliation, on the other hand, involves using products that contain alpha-hydroxy acids (AHAs), beta-hydroxy acids (BHAs), or other chemical exfoliants to dissolve the bonds between dead skin cells, allowing them to be easily removed from the surface of the skin. Chemical exfoliation can be especially effective for Keratosis Pilaris, as it helps to break down the keratin plugs that contribute to the bumpy texture of KP.

Some effective chemical exfoliants for KP include:

1. Glycolic acid: This AHA is derived from sugar cane and is known for its ability to penetrate deeply into the skin, making it an effective choice for treating KP. Look for products with concentrations of 5-10% glycolic acid, and start with a lower concentration if you have sensitive skin.

2. Lactic acid: Another AHA, lactic acid is derived from milk and is known for its gentle, hydrating properties. It's a good choice for those with dry or sensitive skin, and can be found in concentrations of 5-10% in over-the-counter products.

3. Salicylic acid: This BHA is oil-soluble, meaning it can penetrate deep into the pores to unclog them and break down keratin plugs. It's a good choice for those with oily or acne-prone skin, and can be found in concentrations of 0.5-2% in over-the-counter products.

When incorporating chemical exfoliants into your KP skincare routine, it's important to start slowly and gradually increase the frequency and concentration of the products as your skin adjusts. Begin by using the product once or twice a week, and pay close attention to how your skin reacts. If you experience any redness, irritation, or excessive dryness, scale back on the frequency or concentration of the product.

It's also important to use sunscreen daily when using chemical exfoliants, as they can increase the skin's sensitivity to UV radiation. Look for a broad-spectrum sunscreen with an SPF of at least 30, and apply it liberally to all exposed areas of skin.

By incorporating gentle, effective exfoliation methods into your KP skincare routine, you can help to break down the keratin plugs and dead skin cells that contribute to the bumpy texture of KP, leaving your skin smoother, softer, and more even in tone and texture. Just remember to be patient and consistent with your exfoliation routine, and to always listen to your skin's needs and adjust your approach as necessary.

4.3 Moisturizing for Hydration and Barrier Repair

Moisturizing is an essential step in any skincare routine for Keratosis Pilaris, as it helps to hydrate and soften the skin, support the skin's natural barrier function, and reduce the appearance of rough, bumpy texture. When selecting a moisturizer for KP-prone skin, it's important to choose products that are rich in hydrating, nourishing ingredients that can help to soothe and protect the skin.

Some key ingredients to look for in a moisturizer for Keratosis Pilaris include:

1. Urea: This humectant is known for its ability to hydrate and soften the skin, making it an effective choice for managing KP. Look for products with concentrations of 2-10% urea, depending on the severity of your KP and the sensitivity of your skin.

2. Ceramides: These lipid molecules help to support the skin's natural barrier function, preventing moisture loss and protecting the skin from environmental stressors. Look for products that contain ceramides, as well as other barrier-supporting ingredients like cholesterol and fatty acids.

3. Hyaluronic acid: This humectant can hold up to 1000 times its weight in water, making it an excellent choice for hydrating and plumping the skin. Look for products that contain hyaluronic acid, as well as other hydrating ingredients like glycerin and aloe vera.

4. Niacinamide: Also known as vitamin B3, niacinamide is a multipurpose ingredient that can help to reduce inflammation, improve skin texture, and boost the skin's natural ceramide production. Look for products with concentrations of 2-5% niacinamide for best results.

5. Dimethicone: This silicone-based ingredient forms a protective barrier on the surface of the skin, helping to lock in moisture and prevent water loss. It's a good choice for those with very dry or sensitive skin, as it can help to reduce irritation and soothe the skin.

Some moisturizer options that may be suitable for those with Keratosis Pilaris include:

- CeraVe SA Lotion for Rough & Bumpy Skin
   - AmLactin Daily Moisturizing Body Lotion
   - Eucerin Roughness Relief Lotion

- Gold Bond Ultimate Rough & Bumpy Skin Daily Therapy Cream
- Dermadoctor KP Duty Dermatologist Formulated Body Scrub

When applying moisturizer to KP-prone skin, it's important to use gentle, upward strokes and to avoid rubbing or scrubbing the skin, which can cause further irritation. Apply the moisturizer liberally to all affected areas, including the upper arms, thighs, and buttocks, and be sure to moisturize immediately after cleansing or exfoliating to help lock in hydration.

In addition to using a hydrating, nourishing moisturizer, there are other steps you can take to support the health and hydration of your skin:

1. Avoid hot showers and baths: Hot water can strip the skin of its natural oils, leading to dryness and irritation. Instead, use lukewarm water and limit your shower or bath time to 10-15 minutes.

2. Use a humidifier: Dry indoor air can exacerbate KP symptoms, so consider using a humidifier to add moisture to the air and keep your skin hydrated.

3. Drink plenty of water: Staying hydrated from the inside out can help to keep your skin looking and feeling its best. Aim to drink at least 8 glasses of water per day, and more if you're exercising or spending time in hot, dry conditions.

By incorporating a hydrating, nourishing moisturizer into your KP skincare routine and taking steps to support the overall health and hydration of your skin, you can help to reduce the appearance of rough, bumpy texture and improve the overall look and feel of your skin. Remember, consistency is key when it comes to managing KP, so be sure to stick with your moisturizing routine even if you don't see immediate results. With time and patience, you can achieve smoother, softer, more comfortable skin.

CHAPTER 5

Topical Treatments for Keratosis Pilaris: Over-the-Counter and Prescription Options

5.1 Alpha-Hydroxy Acids (AHAs) and Beta-Hydroxy Acids (BHAs)

Alpha-hydroxy acids (AHAs) and beta-hydroxy acids (BHAs) are two classes of chemical exfoliants that can be effective in managing the symptoms of Keratosis Pilaris (KP). These ingredients work by breaking down the bonds between dead skin cells, allowing them to be easily removed from the surface of the skin. This process helps to unclog hair follicles, reduce the buildup of keratin, and improve the overall texture and appearance of KP-affected skin.

AHAs, such as glycolic acid and lactic acid, are water-soluble acids that are derived from natural sources like sugar cane and milk. They work primarily on the surface of the skin, making them a good choice for those with dry or sensitive skin. Glycolic acid, in particular, is known for its ability to penetrate deeply into the skin, making it an effective choice for treating KP. Look for products with concentrations of 5-10% glycolic acid, and start with a lower concentration if you have sensitive skin.

Lactic acid, on the other hand, is a gentler AHA that is known for its hydrating properties. It's a good choice for those with dry or sensitive skin, and can be found in concentrations of 5-10% in over-the-counter products. Lactic acid works by breaking down keratin plugs and promoting cell turnover, leading to smoother, more even-toned skin.

BHAs, such as salicylic acid, are oil-soluble acids that can penetrate deep into the pores to unclog them and break down keratin plugs. Salicylic acid is a good choice for those with oily or acne-prone skin, and can be found in concentrations of 0.5-2% in over-the-counter products. It works by dissolving the bonds between dead skin cells, allowing them to be easily removed from the surface of the skin.

When incorporating AHAs or BHAs into your KP skincare routine, it's important to start slowly and gradually increase the frequency and concentration of the products as your skin adjusts. Begin by using the product once or twice a week, and pay close attention to how your skin reacts. If you experience any redness, irritation, or excessive dryness, scale back on the frequency or concentration of the product.

It's also important to use sunscreen daily when using AHAs or BHAs, as they can increase the skin's sensitivity to UV radiation. Look for a broad-spectrum sunscreen with an SPF of at least 30, and apply it liberally to all exposed areas of skin.

Some over-the-counter products that contain AHAs or BHAs and may be effective for managing KP include:

- Paula's Choice Weightless Body Treatment 2% BHA
    - CeraVe SA Lotion for Rough & Bumpy Skin
    - AmLactin Daily Moisturizing Body Lotion
    - Glytone Exfoliating Body Lotion
    - Eucerin Roughness Relief Lotion

5.2 Urea and Lactic Acid Creams

Urea and lactic acid are two ingredients that are commonly found in over-the-counter creams and lotions for managing Keratosis Pilaris. These ingredients work by hydrating and softening the skin, breaking down keratin plugs, and promoting cell turnover, leading to smoother, more even-toned skin.

Urea is a humectant that occurs naturally in the skin, where it helps to keep the skin hydrated and soft. When applied topically, urea can help to break down the keratin plugs that contribute to the bumpy texture of KP, while also providing deep hydration to the skin. Look for products with concentrations of 2-10% urea, depending on the severity of your KP and the sensitivity of your skin.

Lactic acid, as mentioned earlier, is an alpha-hydroxy acid (AHA) that is derived from milk. It works by breaking down the bonds between dead skin cells, allowing them to be easily removed from the surface of the skin. Lactic acid is known for its gentle, hydrating properties, making it a good choice for those with dry or sensitive skin. Look for products with concentrations of 5-10% lactic acid for best results.

When using urea or lactic acid creams for KP, it's important to apply them consistently and as directed. Most products should be applied once or twice daily, depending on the severity of your KP and the sensitivity of your skin. Be sure to moisturize thoroughly after applying the cream, as this will help to lock in hydration and prevent dryness or irritation.

It's also important to be patient when using urea or lactic acid creams for KP, as it may take several weeks or even months to see noticeable improvements in the texture and appearance of your skin. Stick with your treatment plan, even if you don't see immediate results, and be sure to follow up with your dermatologist if you have any concerns or questions.

Some over-the-counter products that contain urea or lactic acid and may be effective for managing KP include:

- Eucerin Roughness Relief Lotion (contains urea and lactic acid)
   - AmLactin Daily Moisturizing Body Lotion (contains lactic acid)
   - CeraVe SA Lotion for Rough & Bumpy Skin (contains lactic acid and salicylic acid)
   - Excipial 10% Urea Hydrating Healing Lotion
   - Lac-Hydrin Five Moisturizing Lotion (contains lactic acid)

5.3 Retinoids and Vitamin D Analogs

Retinoids and vitamin D analogs are two classes of prescription medications that can be effective in managing the symptoms of Keratosis Pilaris. These medications work by regulating cell turnover, reducing inflammation, and improving the overall texture and appearance of KP-affected skin.

Retinoids are a class of medications that are derived from vitamin A. They work by increasing cell turnover, which helps to unclog hair follicles and reduce the buildup of keratin. Retinoids also have anti-inflammatory properties, which can help to reduce redness and irritation associated with KP.

There are several types of retinoids that may be prescribed for KP, including:

- Tretinoin (Retin-A)
   - Adapalene (Differin)
   - Tazarotene (Tazorac)

These medications are typically applied topically, in the form of creams, gels, or lotions. They should be used as directed by your dermatologist, and it's important to start with a lower concentration and gradually increase as tolerated, to minimize the risk of irritation or dryness.

Vitamin D analogs, such as calcipotriene (Dovonex), are another class of prescription medications that can be effective in managing KP. These medications work by regulating cell growth and differentiation, which helps to reduce the buildup of keratin and improve the overall texture of the skin.

Vitamin D analogs are typically applied topically, in the form of creams, ointments, or solutions. They should be used as directed by your dermatologist, and it's important to follow up regularly to monitor for any side effects or adverse reactions.

When using retinoids or vitamin D analogs for KP, it's important to use them consistently and as directed. It may take several weeks or even months to see noticeable improvements in the texture and appearance of your skin, so it's important to be patient and stick with your treatment plan.

It's also important to use sunscreen daily when using retinoids or vitamin D analogs, as these medications can increase the skin's sensitivity to UV radiation. Look for a broad-spectrum sunscreen with an SPF of at least 30, and apply it liberally to all exposed areas of skin.

In addition to using retinoids or vitamin D analogs, there are other steps you can take to manage KP and support the overall health of your skin:

1. Use a gentle, fragrance-free cleanser to avoid irritating the skin
2. Moisturize regularly with a thick, emollient cream or ointment to lock in hydration and prevent dryness
3. Avoid hot showers or baths, which can strip the skin of its natural oils and cause irritation
4. Use humidifiers to add moisture to the air, especially during dry winter months
5. Wear loose, breathable clothing to avoid irritating the skin
6. Avoid picking or scratching at KP bumps, as this can cause further irritation and inflammation

By working closely with your dermatologist and incorporating a combination of prescription medications, over-the-counter treatments, and lifestyle modifications, you can effectively manage the symptoms of Keratosis Pilaris and achieve smoother, more even-toned skin. Remember, everyone's skin is unique, so it may take some trial and error to find the treatment plan that works best for you. Be patient, stay consistent, and don't hesitate to reach out to your dermatologist if you have any concerns or questions along the way.

CHAPTER 6

In-Office Treatments for Keratosis Pilaris: Professional Procedures

6.1 Chemical Peels

Chemical peels are a popular in-office treatment for Keratosis Pilaris (KP) that involve the application of a chemical solution to the skin, causing it to exfoliate and eventually peel off. This process helps to unclog hair follicles, reduce the buildup of keratin, and improve the overall texture and appearance of KP-affected skin.

There are several types of chemical peels that may be used to treat KP, including:

1. Glycolic acid peels: Glycolic acid is an alpha-hydroxy acid (AHA) that is derived from sugar cane. It works by breaking down the bonds between dead skin cells, allowing them to be easily removed from the surface of the skin. Glycolic acid peels typically range in concentration from 20-70%, depending on the severity of the KP and the patient's skin type.

2. Salicylic acid peels: Salicylic acid is a beta-hydroxy acid (BHA) that is oil-soluble, allowing it to penetrate deep into the pores and break down keratin plugs. Salicylic acid peels typically range in concentration from 20-30% and are a good option for those with oily or acne-prone skin.

3. Lactic acid peels: Lactic acid is another type of AHA that is derived from milk. It is known for its gentle, hydrating properties and is a good option for those with dry or sensitive skin. Lactic acid peels typically range in concentration from 20-50%.

During a chemical peel treatment for KP, the skin will first be cleansed and prepped. The chemical solution will then be applied to the affected areas and left on for a specific amount of time, typically ranging from 3-10 minutes, depending on the type and strength of the peel. The solution will then be neutralized and removed, and a moisturizer and sunscreen will be applied to the skin.

After the treatment, the skin may be red, sensitive, and may even peel or flake for several days. It's important to follow the post-treatment instructions provided by your dermatologist, which may include avoiding sun exposure, using gentle skincare products, and moisturizing regularly to support the healing process.

The number of chemical peel treatments needed for KP will vary depending on the severity of the condition and the individual's response to treatment. Most people will need a series of treatments, spaced several weeks apart, to achieve optimal results. It's important to work closely with your dermatologist to develop a treatment plan that is tailored to your specific needs and goals.

6.2 Microdermabrasion and Dermabrasion

Microdermabrasion and dermabrasion are two types of mechanical exfoliation treatments that can be effective in managing the symptoms of Keratosis Pilaris. These treatments work by physically removing the top layer of dead skin cells, unclogging hair follicles, and promoting cell turnover, resulting in smoother, more even-toned skin.

Microdermabrasion is a minimally invasive treatment that uses a handheld device to spray fine crystals onto the skin, gently exfoliating the surface. The device then suctions away the crystals and exfoliated skin cells, leaving the skin smooth and refreshed. Microdermabrasion is typically well-tolerated and requires little to no downtime, making it a popular choice for those with mild to moderate KP.

During a microdermabrasion treatment for KP, the skin will first be cleansed and prepped. The handheld device will then be passed over the affected areas, typically for several passes, depending on the severity of the KP and the individual's tolerance. After the treatment, a moisturizer and sunscreen will be applied to the skin.

Dermabrasion, on the other hand, is a more aggressive form of mechanical exfoliation that uses a rapidly rotating device to sand down the top layer of skin. This treatment is typically reserved for more severe cases of KP and is performed under local anesthesia. Dermabrasion can cause significant redness, swelling, and scabbing, and may require several weeks of downtime for healing.

During a dermabrasion treatment for KP, the skin will first be cleansed and prepped, and a local anesthetic will be applied to minimize discomfort. The rotating device will then be passed over the affected areas, carefully removing the top layer of skin. After the treatment, a moisturizer and protective ointment will be applied to the skin, and the patient will be given specific instructions for post-treatment care.

As with chemical peels, the number of microdermabrasion or dermabrasion treatments needed for KP will vary depending on the severity of the condition and the individual's response to treatment. Most people will need a series of treatments, spaced several weeks apart, to achieve optimal results.

It's important to note that while microdermabrasion and dermabrasion can be effective in managing KP, they are not a cure for the condition. KP is a chronic skin disorder that may require ongoing maintenance treatments to keep symptoms under control. It's important to work closely with your dermatologist to develop a long-term treatment plan that includes a combination of in-office treatments, at-home skincare, and lifestyle modifications.

6.3 Laser and Light Therapies

Laser and light therapies are advanced in-office treatments that can be effective in managing the symptoms of Keratosis Pilaris. These treatments work by targeting specific structures within the skin, such as hair follicles or pigment cells, to reduce inflammation, promote cell turnover, and improve the overall texture and appearance of KP-affected skin.

There are several types of laser and light therapies that may be used to treat KP, including:

1. Pulsed dye laser (PDL): PDL is a type of laser that uses a specific wavelength of light to target blood vessels in the skin. This can help to reduce redness and inflammation associated with KP, as well as improve the overall texture of the skin. PDL treatments are typically well-tolerated and require little to no downtime.

2. Intense pulsed light (IPL): IPL is a type of light therapy that uses a broad spectrum of light to target pigment cells and blood vessels in the skin. This can help to reduce redness, even out skin tone, and improve the overall texture of KP-affected skin. IPL treatments are typically well-tolerated and require little to no downtime.

3. Fractional laser resurfacing: Fractional laser resurfacing is a type of laser treatment that creates microscopic wounds in the skin, stimulating collagen production and promoting cell turnover. This can help to improve the overall

texture and appearance of KP-affected skin, as well as reduce the appearance of scarring or hyperpigmentation. Fractional laser resurfacing treatments typically require several days to a week of downtime for healing.

During a laser or light therapy treatment for KP, the skin will first be cleansed and prepped. A topical anesthetic may be applied to minimize discomfort during the treatment. The laser or light device will then be passed over the affected areas, typically for several passes, depending on the severity of the KP and the individual's tolerance. After the treatment, a moisturizer and sunscreen will be applied to the skin.

As with other in-office treatments for KP, the number of laser or light therapy treatments needed will vary depending on the severity of the condition and the individual's response to treatment. Most people will need a series of treatments, spaced several weeks apart, to achieve optimal results.

While laser and light therapies can be highly effective in managing KP, they do come with some risks and potential side effects. These may include redness, swelling, bruising, or changes in skin pigmentation. It's important to work closely with a qualified dermatologist who has experience in using these treatments for KP, and to carefully follow all pre- and post-treatment instructions to minimize the risk of complications.

In addition to in-office treatments, there are several other strategies that can help to manage the symptoms of KP and improve the overall health and appearance of the skin. These may include:

1. Using gentle, fragrance-free skincare products that are designed for sensitive skin
2. Avoiding harsh scrubs or exfoliants that can irritate the skin
3. Moisturizing regularly with a thick, emollient cream or ointment to lock in hydration and prevent dryness

4. Using humidifiers to add moisture to the air, especially during dry winter months
5. Wearing loose, breathable clothing to avoid irritating the skin
6. Avoiding hot showers or baths, which can strip the skin of its natural oils and cause irritation

By working closely with a qualified dermatologist and developing a personalized treatment plan that includes a combination of in-office treatments, at-home skincare, and lifestyle modifications, most people with KP can achieve significant improvements in the texture and appearance of their skin. With patience, persistence, and a commitment to self-care, it is possible to manage the symptoms of KP and feel confident and comfortable in your own skin.

CHAPTER 7

Natural Remedies and Home Treatments for Keratosis Pilaris

7.1 Herbal and Plant-Based Remedies

In addition to professional treatments and over-the-counter products, many people with Keratosis Pilaris (KP) find relief through the use of natural, herbal, and plant-based remedies. These remedies can be used alone or in conjunction with other treatments to help soothe and nourish the skin, reduce inflammation, and promote healing.

Some of the most popular herbal and plant-based remedies for KP include:

1. Aloe vera: Aloe vera is a succulent plant that is well-known for its soothing, anti-inflammatory properties. The clear gel found inside the leaves of the aloe vera plant can be applied directly to KP-affected skin to help reduce redness, itching, and irritation. Aloe vera is also rich in vitamins and minerals that can help to nourish and moisturize the skin.

2. Coconut oil: Coconut oil is a natural, plant-based oil that is rich in fatty acids and antioxidants. When applied topically to KP-affected skin, coconut oil can help to moisturize and soften rough, dry patches, as well as reduce inflammation and redness. Coconut oil is also naturally antimicrobial, which can help to prevent the growth of bacteria and other microorganisms on the skin.

3. Tea tree oil: Tea tree oil is an essential oil derived from the leaves of the tea tree plant. It has natural antiseptic, anti-inflammatory, and antimicrobial properties that can help to soothe and heal KP-affected skin. Tea tree oil should always be diluted with a carrier oil, such as coconut or jojoba oil, before being applied to the skin to prevent irritation.

4. Apple cider vinegar: Apple cider vinegar is a natural, acidic liquid that can help to exfoliate and balance the pH of the skin. When applied topically to KP-affected areas, apple cider vinegar can help to unclog hair follicles, reduce inflammation, and promote cell turnover. To use apple cider vinegar for KP, mix equal parts water and vinegar and apply the solution to the skin using a cotton ball or pad. Rinse off after several minutes and follow with a moisturizer.

5. Oatmeal: Oatmeal is a natural, gentle exfoliant that can help to soothe and nourish KP-affected skin. Colloidal oatmeal, which is a finely ground form of oatmeal that is suspended in liquid, can be added to bathwater or used as a paste to help reduce inflammation, itching, and dryness. Oatmeal is also rich in antioxidants and vitamins that can help to promote healthy skin.

When using herbal and plant-based remedies for KP, it's important to choose high-quality, pure ingredients and to patch test any new products before applying them to larger areas of the skin. It's also important to be patient and consistent with natural remedies, as they may take longer to produce visible results than traditional treatments.

In addition to topical remedies, some people with KP find relief through the use of oral herbal supplements, such as evening primrose oil or omega-3 fatty acids. These supplements can help to reduce inflammation and promote healthy skin from the inside out. However, it's important to talk to your dermatologist or a qualified healthcare provider before starting any new supplements, as they may interact with other medications or have potential side effects.

7.2 DIY Scrubs and Masks

In addition to herbal and plant-based remedies, many people with Keratosis Pilaris find relief through the use of homemade scrubs and masks. These DIY treatments can help to exfoliate and nourish the skin, reduce inflammation, and promote cell turnover, all of which can improve the appearance and texture of KP-affected skin.

Some simple and effective DIY scrubs and masks for KP include:

1. Sugar scrub: Sugar is a natural, gentle exfoliant that can help to unclog hair follicles and remove dead skin cells. To make a sugar scrub for KP, mix equal parts sugar and a carrier oil, such as coconut or jojoba oil, until a paste forms. Gently massage the scrub onto damp skin in a circular motion, paying extra attention to rough, bumpy areas. Rinse off with warm water and follow with a moisturizer.

2. Honey and oatmeal mask: Honey is a natural humectant that can help to moisturize and soften the skin, while oatmeal is a gentle exfoliant that can help to soothe and nourish. To make a honey and oatmeal mask for KP, mix equal parts honey and colloidal oatmeal until a paste forms. Apply the mixture to clean, damp skin and leave on for 10-15 minutes before rinsing off with warm water.

3. Avocado and yogurt mask: Avocado is rich in healthy fats and vitamins that can help to nourish and moisturize the skin, while yogurt contains lactic acid, a gentle alpha-hydroxy acid that can help to exfoliate and soften rough, dry patches. To make an avocado and yogurt mask for KP, mash half an avocado and mix it with 1/4 cup of plain, unsweetened yogurt. Apply the mixture to clean, damp skin and leave on for 10-15 minutes before rinsing off with warm water.

4. Baking soda scrub: Baking soda is a gentle, alkaline exfoliant that can

help to unclog hair follicles and remove dead skin cells. To make a baking soda scrub for KP, mix equal parts baking soda and water until a paste forms. Gently massage the scrub onto damp skin in a circular motion, paying extra attention to rough, bumpy areas. Rinse off with warm water and follow with a moisturizer.

When using DIY scrubs and masks for KP, it's important to be gentle and to avoid over-exfoliating the skin, which can cause irritation and inflammation. It's also important to patch test any new ingredients before applying them to larger areas of the skin, as some people may be sensitive or allergic to certain ingredients.

In addition to scrubs and masks, some people with KP find relief through the use of homemade moisturizers and balms. These products can help to soothe and hydrate the skin, as well as protect it from environmental stressors. Some simple and effective DIY moisturizers for KP include:

1. Whipped shea butter: Shea butter is a rich, nourishing butter that can help to moisturize and soften rough, dry skin. To make whipped shea butter for KP, simply whip room-temperature shea butter with a hand mixer until it becomes light and fluffy. You can also add a few drops of your favorite essential oil for added fragrance and benefits.

2. Coconut oil balm: Coconut oil is a natural, plant-based oil that is rich in fatty acids and antioxidants. To make a coconut oil balm for KP, simply melt 1/2 cup of coconut oil with 1/4 cup of beeswax pellets in a double boiler. Pour the mixture into a jar and let it cool and solidify before using.

By incorporating DIY scrubs, masks, and moisturizers into your KP skincare routine, you can help to nourish and soothe your skin, as well as improve its overall texture and appearance. Just remember to be patient, consistent, and gentle with your skin, and to always listen to your body and adjust your routine as needed.

7.3 Lifestyle Changes for Skin Health

While topical treatments and remedies can be effective in managing the symptoms of Keratosis Pilaris, making certain lifestyle changes can also have a significant impact on the overall health and appearance of your skin. By adopting healthy habits and making simple modifications to your daily routine, you can help to support your skin from the inside out and improve the effectiveness of your KP treatment plan.

Some lifestyle changes that can benefit people with KP include:

1. Staying hydrated: Drinking plenty of water and other hydrating fluids throughout the day can help to keep your skin moisturized and supple from the inside out. Aim to drink at least 8-10 glasses of water per day, and more if you are physically active or live in a dry climate.

2. Eating a healthy diet: A diet that is rich in fruits, vegetables, whole grains, and lean proteins can provide your skin with the nutrients it needs to stay healthy and resilient. Foods that are particularly beneficial for skin health include those that are high in antioxidants, such as berries, leafy greens, and nuts, as well as those that are rich in healthy fats, such as avocados, fatty fish, and olive oil.

3. Managing stress: Chronic stress can take a toll on your skin, leading to inflammation, breakouts, and other issues. To help manage stress and support healthy skin, try incorporating stress-reducing activities into your daily routine, such as meditation, deep breathing, or yoga. You can also try to prioritize self-care activities that help you to relax and unwind, such as taking a warm bath, reading a book, or spending time in nature.

4. Getting enough sleep: Sleep is essential for overall health and well-being, including the health of your skin. During sleep, your body works to repair and regenerate cells, including skin cells. Aim to get 7-9 hours of quality sleep

per night, and try to establish a consistent sleep schedule to help regulate your body's natural rhythms.

5. Exercising regularly: Regular physical activity can help to improve circulation, boost immune function, and reduce stress, all of which can benefit the health of your skin. Aim to get at least 30 minutes of moderate-intensity exercise most days of the week, such as brisk walking, cycling, or swimming.

6. Avoiding hot showers and baths: While a hot shower or bath can feel soothing, the heat and steam can actually strip your skin of its natural oils, leading to dryness and irritation. Instead, try to keep your showers and baths lukewarm and limit them to 10-15 minutes at a time. Afterward, be sure to moisturize your skin while it is still damp to help lock in hydration.

7. Wearing loose, breathable clothing: Tight, restrictive clothing can rub against your skin and cause irritation, especially in areas where KP is present. Instead, opt for loose, breathable clothing made from natural fibers, such as cotton or bamboo, which can help to reduce friction and allow your skin to breathe.

8. Protecting your skin from the sun: While a little bit of sun exposure can be beneficial for vitamin D production, too much sun can damage your skin and exacerbate KP symptoms. To protect your skin, try to limit your time in direct sunlight, especially during peak hours (10am-4pm), and always wear a broad-spectrum sunscreen with an SPF of at least 30 when spending time outdoors.

By making these lifestyle changes and incorporating them into your daily routine, you can help to support the health and resilience of your skin, as well as improve the effectiveness of your KP treatment plan. Remember, everyone's skin is different, and what works for one person may not work for another. Be patient, listen to your body, and don't hesitate to seek guidance from a qualified healthcare provider if you have any concerns or questions about your skin health.

CHAPTER 8

Keratosis Pilaris and Diet: Nutritional Strategies for Skin Improvement

8.1 Foods to Eat and Avoid

While there is no one-size-fits-all diet for managing Keratosis Pilaris (KP), certain nutritional strategies may help to support skin health and reduce the severity of KP symptoms. By focusing on nutrient-dense, whole foods and limiting processed, inflammatory foods, you can provide your skin with the building blocks it needs to stay healthy and resilient.

Foods to include in a KP-friendly diet:

1. Fatty fish: Fatty fish, such as salmon, mackerel, and sardines, are rich in omega-3 fatty acids, which have anti-inflammatory properties and can help to support skin health. Omega-3s can also help to improve skin hydration and reduce dryness, which is a common issue for people with KP.

2. Leafy greens: Leafy greens, such as spinach, kale, and Swiss chard, are packed with vitamins and minerals that are essential for skin health, including vitamin A, vitamin C, and folate. These nutrients can help to support collagen production, protect against oxidative stress, and promote healthy cell turnover.

3. Berries: Berries, such as blueberries, raspberries, and strawberries, are high in antioxidants, which can help to protect the skin from damage caused by free radicals. Antioxidants can also help to reduce inflammation and support healthy collagen production.

4. Nuts and seeds: Nuts and seeds, such as almonds, walnuts, and flaxseeds, are rich in healthy fats, vitamins, and minerals that can support skin health. For example, almonds are a good source of vitamin E, which can help to protect the skin from UV damage and reduce inflammation.

5. Avocados: Avocados are rich in healthy monounsaturated fats, as well as vitamins C, E, and K. These nutrients can help to moisturize the skin from the inside out, as well as protect against oxidative stress and inflammation.

6. Sweet potatoes: Sweet potatoes are an excellent source of beta-carotene, which the body converts into vitamin A. Vitamin A is essential for healthy skin cell turnover and can help to reduce the buildup of keratin that contributes to KP.

Foods to limit or avoid:

1. Processed and refined carbohydrates: Processed and refined carbohydrates, such as white bread, pasta, and sugary snacks, can cause rapid spikes in blood sugar, which can lead to inflammation and contribute to skin issues like KP. Instead, opt for whole-grain, fiber-rich carbohydrates that are digested more slowly and have a lower glycemic index.

2. Dairy products: Some people with KP find that consuming dairy products, such as milk, cheese, and yogurt, can exacerbate their symptoms. This may be due to the hormones and growth factors present in dairy, which can stimulate oil production and contribute to inflammation. If you suspect that dairy may be a trigger for your KP, try eliminating it from your diet for a few weeks to see if your symptoms improve.

3. Fried and greasy foods: Fried and greasy foods, such as french fries, fried chicken, and pizza, are high in unhealthy fats and can contribute to inflammation and skin issues. Instead, opt for baked, grilled, or roasted foods that are cooked with healthy fats, such as olive oil or avocado oil.

4. Alcohol: Alcohol can dehydrate the skin and contribute to inflammation, which can worsen KP symptoms. If you do choose to drink alcohol, be sure to stay hydrated by drinking plenty of water and limiting your intake to one or two drinks per day.

5. Spicy foods: Some people with KP find that consuming spicy foods, such as hot peppers or curry, can cause flushing and irritation in their skin. If you notice that spicy foods seem to trigger your KP symptoms, try limiting or avoiding them to see if your skin improves.

By focusing on nutrient-dense, whole foods and limiting processed, inflammatory foods, you can support the overall health and resilience of your skin. However, it's important to remember that diet is just one piece of the puzzle when it comes to managing KP. A holistic approach that includes a consistent skincare routine, lifestyle modifications, and guidance from a qualified healthcare provider is often the most effective way to manage KP symptoms and improve the overall health and appearance of your skin.

8.2 Nutritional Supplements for Skin Health

In addition to following a nutrient-dense, whole-foods diet, some people with Keratosis Pilaris (KP) may benefit from taking certain nutritional supplements to support skin health. While supplements should never be used as a replacement for a healthy diet and lifestyle, they can help to fill in nutritional gaps and provide targeted support for specific skin concerns.

Some nutritional supplements that may be beneficial for people with KP include:

1. Omega-3 fatty acids: Omega-3 fatty acids, such as those found in fish oil supplements, can help to reduce inflammation and support skin hydration. Some studies have also suggested that omega-3s may help to improve the overall texture and appearance of the skin.

2. Vitamin D: Vitamin D is essential for skin health and plays a role in regulating skin cell growth and differentiation. Some studies have found that people with KP may be more likely to have low levels of vitamin D, and that supplementing with vitamin D may help to improve KP symptoms.

3. Vitamin A: Vitamin A is important for healthy skin cell turnover and can help to reduce the buildup of keratin that contributes to KP. While vitamin A can be obtained through the diet in the form of beta-carotene, some people may benefit from taking a vitamin A supplement, particularly if they have a deficiency.

4. Zinc: Zinc is a mineral that plays a key role in skin health, including wound healing and inflammation control. Some studies have suggested that people with KP may have lower levels of zinc in their skin, and that supplementing with zinc may help to improve KP symptoms.

5. Probiotics: Probiotics are beneficial bacteria that live in the gut and play a role in immune function and skin health. Some studies have suggested that taking a probiotic supplement may help to reduce inflammation and improve the overall health and appearance of the skin.

When considering nutritional supplements for KP, it's important to talk to your healthcare provider first. Some supplements can interact with medications or have side effects, and it's important to make sure that they are safe and appropriate for your individual needs. Your healthcare provider can also help you to determine the right dosage and form of supplement to take, based on your age, health status, and other factors.

It's also important to choose high-quality supplements from reputable brands, and to store them properly to ensure their potency and safety. Look for supplements that have been third-party tested for purity and potency, and that are free from artificial additives, fillers, and contaminants.

While nutritional supplements can be a helpful addition to a KP management plan, they should never be relied upon as the sole treatment for KP. A holistic approach that includes a consistent skincare routine, healthy diet and lifestyle habits, and guidance from a qualified healthcare provider is often the most effective way to manage KP symptoms and support overall skin health.

8.3 Hydration and Its Impact on Keratosis Pilaris

Proper hydration is essential for overall health and well-being, and it plays a particularly important role in skin health. When the body is well-hydrated, the skin is better able to maintain its moisture balance, elasticity, and resilience. Conversely, when the body is dehydrated, the skin can become dry, flaky, and more prone to irritation and inflammation.

For people with Keratosis Pilaris (KP), staying properly hydrated is especially important. Dry, dehydrated skin can exacerbate KP symptoms, making the bumps and rough patches more noticeable and uncomfortable. Drinking plenty of water and other hydrating fluids throughout the day can help to keep the skin moisturized and supple from the inside out, which can help to reduce the severity of KP symptoms.

In addition to drinking water, there are other ways to support skin hydration and improve KP symptoms:

1. Eat hydrating foods: Many fruits and vegetables have a high water content and can help to hydrate the body from the inside out. Some particularly hydrating options include watermelon, cucumbers, zucchini, and leafy greens.

2. Use a humidifier: Dry indoor air can sap moisture from the skin, exacerbating KP symptoms. Using a humidifier, especially in the bedroom, can help to add moisture back into the air and prevent the skin from becoming too dry.

3. Limit caffeine and alcohol: Both caffeine and alcohol can have a diuretic effect, meaning that they can increase urine production and lead to dehydration. While it's okay to enjoy these beverages in moderation, it's important to balance them out with plenty of water and other hydrating fluids.

4. Use a gentle, non-drying cleanser: Harsh, drying cleansers can strip the skin of its natural oils and lead to dehydration and irritation. Choose a gentle, non-foaming cleanser that is designed for sensitive skin, and avoid hot water, which can further dry out the skin.

5. Moisturize regularly: Applying a thick, emollient moisturizer to damp skin can help to lock in hydration and prevent moisture loss. Look for moisturizers that contain humectants, such as glycerin or hyaluronic acid, which can help to draw moisture into the skin.

6. Protect the skin from the elements: Exposure to wind, cold, and sun can all contribute to skin dehydration and irritation. Protect the skin by wearing loose, breathable clothing, using a broad-spectrum sunscreen, and limiting time spent in harsh weather conditions.

By prioritizing hydration and taking steps to support skin moisture balance, people with KP can help to reduce the severity of their symptoms and improve the overall health and appearance of their skin. However, it's important to remember that hydration is just one piece of the puzzle when it comes to managing KP. A holistic approach that includes a consistent skincare routine, healthy diet and lifestyle habits, and guidance from a qualified healthcare provider is often the most effective way to manage KP symptoms and support overall skin health.

In conclusion, while there is no one-size-fits-all approach to managing Keratosis Pilaris through diet and nutrition, making certain dietary and lifestyle modifications can be a helpful complement to a comprehensive KP treatment plan. By focusing on nutrient-dense, whole foods, staying properly hydrated, and considering targeted nutritional supplements under the guidance of a healthcare provider, people with KP can support the overall health and resilience of their skin and potentially reduce the severity of their symptoms. However, it's important to remember that diet and nutrition are just one aspect of a holistic approach to managing KP, and that a consistent skincare routine, healthy lifestyle habits, and guidance from a qualified healthcare provider are also essential for achieving and maintaining healthy, comfortable skin.

CHAPTER 9

Keratosis Pilaris in Different Life Stages: Children, Teenagers, and Adults

Keratosis Pilaris (KP) is a common skin condition that can affect people of all ages, from infants to adults. While the basic characteristics of KP remain the same across different life stages, there are some unique considerations and challenges that may arise depending on an individual's age and stage of life. In this chapter, we'll explore how KP can manifest and be managed in children, teenagers, and adults.

9.1 Caring for Children with Keratosis Pilaris

Keratosis Pilaris can develop in children as young as infants, and it's estimated that up to 50-80% of children may have some degree of KP. In children, KP often appears as small, rough, pink or red bumps on the cheeks, upper arms, thighs, or buttocks. While KP is not harmful or contagious, it can be itchy or uncomfortable for some children, and may cause emotional distress if the child feels self-conscious about their skin.

When caring for a child with KP, it's important to take a gentle, patient approach that focuses on soothing and moisturizing the skin. Some tips for managing KP in children include:

1. Use a gentle, fragrance-free cleanser: Children's skin is often more delicate

and sensitive than adult skin, so it's important to use a mild, non-irritating cleanser that won't strip the skin of its natural oils. Look for a cleanser that is specifically designed for sensitive skin, and avoid harsh scrubs or exfoliants.

2. Moisturize regularly: Keeping the skin well-hydrated is key to managing KP in children. Apply a thick, emollient moisturizer to damp skin after bathing, and reapply as needed throughout the day. Look for moisturizers that contain ingredients like glycerin, shea butter, or ceramides, which can help to soothe and protect the skin.

3. Avoid hot baths and showers: Hot water can dry out and irritate the skin, exacerbating KP symptoms. Keep bath and shower water lukewarm, and limit bathing time to 10-15 minutes to prevent over-drying the skin.

4. Use a humidifier: Dry indoor air can contribute to skin dryness and irritation. Running a humidifier in your child's room can help to add moisture back into the air and keep the skin hydrated.

5. Dress in soft, breathable fabrics: Rough, irritating fabrics can rub against the skin and exacerbate KP symptoms. Dress your child in soft, breathable fabrics like cotton or bamboo, and avoid tight or restrictive clothing that can trap heat and moisture.

6. Be patient and consistent: KP can be a stubborn condition, and it may take time and consistent care to see improvement in your child's skin. Be patient and persistent with your child's skincare routine, and celebrate small victories along the way.

It's also important to talk to your child about their KP in an age-appropriate way, and to emphasize that the condition is common, treatable, and not a reflection of their worth or attractiveness. If your child is experiencing significant discomfort or distress related to their KP, don't hesitate to talk to your pediatrician or a pediatric dermatologist for additional guidance and support.

9.2 Managing Keratosis Pilaris During Puberty and Adolescence

Puberty and adolescence can be challenging times for many young people, and the hormonal changes and growth spurts that occur during this period can sometimes exacerbate Keratosis Pilaris symptoms. As adolescents become more self-aware and self-conscious about their appearance, KP can also take a toll on their self-esteem and body image.

When managing KP during the teenage years, it's important to take a holistic approach that addresses both the physical and emotional aspects of the condition. Some strategies for managing KP in teenagers include:

1. Develop a consistent skincare routine: Encourage your teenager to develop a simple, consistent skincare routine that includes gentle cleansing, exfoliation, and moisturizing. Help them to find products that work well for their skin type and preferences, and encourage them to stick with the routine even if they don't see immediate results.

2. Consider topical treatments: Over-the-counter topical treatments like salicylic acid, lactic acid, or urea cream can be helpful for managing KP symptoms in teenagers. Encourage your teenager to patch test any new products before using them more widely, and to follow the instructions for use carefully.

3. Address nutritional needs: The teenage years are a time of rapid growth and development, and proper nutrition is essential for overall health and well-being. Encourage your teenager to eat a balanced, nutrient-rich diet that includes plenty of fruits, vegetables, lean proteins, and healthy fats. Consider talking to your teenager's doctor about whether nutritional supplements may be appropriate.

4. Encourage healthy lifestyle habits: Healthy lifestyle habits like regular exercise, stress management, and sufficient sleep can all support skin health and overall well-being. Encourage your teenager to find physical activities they enjoy, to practice stress-reducing techniques like deep breathing or meditation, and to prioritize getting enough rest each night.

5. Provide emotional support: The emotional impact of KP can be significant during the teenage years, when many young people are already struggling with self-esteem and body image issues. Provide a listening ear and emotional support for your teenager, and encourage them to talk openly about their feelings and concerns related to their skin. Consider seeking support from a mental health professional if your teenager is experiencing significant distress related to their KP.

6. Be a positive role model: As a parent or caregiver, you can be a powerful role model for your teenager when it comes to self-acceptance and body positivity. Model healthy attitudes towards your own body and appearance, and avoid making negative comments about your own or others' skin or appearance.

Remember, while the teenage years can be a challenging time for managing KP, they are also an opportunity to help your teenager develop lifelong habits of self-care and self-acceptance. By providing support, encouragement, and practical guidance, you can help your teenager navigate this stage of life with confidence and resilience.

9.3 Keratosis Pilaris in Adulthood: Hormonal Influences and Aging Skin

While Keratosis Pilaris is often thought of as a childhood or adolescent condition, many adults continue to experience KP symptoms throughout their lives. In adulthood, hormonal changes and the natural aging process can influence the severity and appearance of KP, and may require adjustments to treatment and management strategies.

Hormonal changes, particularly those related to pregnancy and menopause, can have a significant impact on KP symptoms in adults. During pregnancy, increased levels of hormones like estrogen and progesterone can cause skin changes, including increased dryness, sensitivity, and hyperpigmentation. Some women may find that their KP symptoms worsen during pregnancy, while others may experience a temporary improvement.

Similarly, during menopause, declining levels of estrogen can lead to skin changes like dryness, thinning, and loss of elasticity. These changes can exacerbate KP symptoms and make the skin more prone to irritation and inflammation. Women going through menopause may need to adjust their skincare routine to account for these changes, and may benefit from products that are specifically formulated for mature skin.

In addition to hormonal influences, the natural aging process can also impact the appearance and severity of KP in adults. As we age, our skin tends to become drier, thinner, and less resilient, making it more prone to irritation and damage. Sun exposure, environmental stressors, and lifestyle factors like smoking or poor nutrition can also contribute to premature aging and exacerbate KP symptoms.

When managing KP in adulthood, it's important to take a comprehensive approach that addresses both the physical and emotional aspects of the condition. Some strategies for managing KP in adults include:

1. Adjusting your skincare routine: As your skin changes with age and hormonal fluctuations, you may need to adjust your skincare routine accordingly. Look for products that are specifically formulated for mature or sensitive skin, and that contain ingredients like hyaluronic acid, ceramides, or niacinamide to help support skin hydration and resilience.

2. Protecting your skin from the sun: Sun exposure can exacerbate KP symptoms and contribute to premature aging and hyperpigmentation. Be

diligent about wearing broad-spectrum sunscreen with an SPF of at least 30 every day, and protect your skin with clothing, hats, and shade when possible.

3. Managing stress: Chronic stress can take a toll on the skin, exacerbating inflammation and slowing down healing processes. Practice stress-reducing techniques like deep breathing, meditation, or yoga, and make time for activities that bring you joy and relaxation.

4. Staying hydrated: Drinking plenty of water and eating a diet rich in hydrating fruits and vegetables can help to keep your skin hydrated and healthy from the inside out. Aim to drink at least 8 glasses of water per day, and more if you're exercising or spending time in dry or hot environments.

5. Considering professional treatments: If over-the-counter treatments and lifestyle modifications aren't providing sufficient relief from your KP symptoms, consider talking to a dermatologist about professional treatment options like chemical peels, microdermabrasion, or laser therapy.

6. Focusing on self-care and self-acceptance: As we age, it's natural for our skin to change and develop imperfections. Rather than striving for an unrealistic ideal of perfect skin, focus on practicing self-care and self-acceptance. Celebrate your unique beauty, and prioritize taking care of yourself physically, emotionally, and mentally.

Remember, while managing KP in adulthood can present unique challenges, it's also an opportunity to develop a deeper understanding of your skin and your overall health and well-being. By taking a comprehensive, self-compassionate approach to KP management, you can help to support healthy, resilient skin at any age.

In conclusion, Keratosis Pilaris can present unique challenges and considerations at different stages of life, from childhood to adolescence to adulthood. By taking a developmental approach to KP management, and tailoring treatment strategies to the specific needs and concerns of each life stage, individuals with KP can help to support healthy, comfortable skin throughout their lives. Whether you're caring for a child with KP, supporting a teenager through the challenges of puberty, or navigating the hormonal and aging-related changes of adulthood, remember that patience, consistency, and self-compassion are key to managing this common and treatable skin condition.

CHAPTER 10

Keratosis Pilaris and Associated Conditions: Atopic Dermatitis and More

Keratosis Pilaris (KP) is a skin condition that often occurs in isolation, but it can also be associated with other skin disorders or systemic conditions. Understanding these associations can be important for individuals with KP, as they may require additional or specialized treatment approaches to manage their symptoms effectively. In this chapter, we'll explore some of the most common conditions associated with KP, including atopic dermatitis, ichthyosis vulgaris, and others.

10.1 The Link Between Keratosis Pilaris and Atopic Dermatitis

Atopic dermatitis, also known as eczema, is a chronic inflammatory skin condition that causes dry, itchy, and inflamed skin. It is one of the most common skin disorders associated with Keratosis Pilaris, with some studies suggesting that up to 50% of people with KP also have atopic dermatitis.

The link between KP and atopic dermatitis is thought to be related to a shared genetic and immunological basis. Both conditions are characterized by a dysfunction in the skin barrier, which allows moisture to escape and irritants to penetrate the skin more easily. This dysfunction is thought to be related to mutations in the filaggrin gene, which plays a key role in maintaining the integrity of the skin barrier.

In addition to genetic factors, environmental and lifestyle factors can also contribute to the development and exacerbation of both KP and atopic dermatitis. These may include exposure to irritants or allergens, harsh skincare products, stress, and changes in temperature or humidity.

When managing KP in individuals with atopic dermatitis, it's important to take a gentle, protective approach that focuses on supporting the skin barrier and reducing inflammation. Some strategies may include:

1. Using gentle, fragrance-free cleansers and moisturizers that are specifically formulated for sensitive or eczema-prone skin.
2. Avoiding hot showers or baths, which can strip the skin of its natural oils and exacerbate dryness and irritation.
3. Applying emollient creams or ointments to damp skin to help lock in moisture and protect the skin barrier.
4. Using humidifiers to add moisture to the air, particularly in dry or cold environments.
5. Identifying and avoiding triggers that exacerbate eczema symptoms, such as certain foods, fabrics, or environmental allergens.
6. Considering topical or oral medications, such as corticosteroids or immunomodulators, to help control inflammation and itching.

In some cases, individuals with KP and atopic dermatitis may also benefit from systemic treatments that address the underlying immune dysfunction, such as biologic medications or immunosuppressants. However, these treatments should only be used under the guidance of a qualified healthcare provider, as they can have significant side effects and risks.

10.2 Keratosis Pilaris and Ichthyosis Vulgaris

Ichthyosis vulgaris is a genetic skin disorder characterized by dry, scaly skin that may resemble fish scales. It is caused by mutations in the filaggrin gene, which is also implicated in the development of Keratosis Pilaris and atopic dermatitis.

While not all individuals with ichthyosis vulgaris will develop KP, the two conditions often co-occur, particularly in more severe cases of ichthyosis. In fact, some studies suggest that up to 70% of individuals with moderate to severe ichthyosis vulgaris also have KP.

When managing KP in individuals with ichthyosis vulgaris, it's important to focus on intensive moisturization and gentle exfoliation to help improve skin texture and reduce the buildup of scales. Some strategies may include:

1. Using thick, emollient creams or ointments that contain ingredients like urea, lactic acid, or ceramides to help soften and moisturize the skin.
2. Applying moisturizers to damp skin immediately after bathing or showering to help lock in hydration.
3. Using gentle, non-abrasive exfoliants like alpha-hydroxy acids or salicylic acid to help loosen and remove scales.
4. Taking lukewarm baths or showers and limiting bathing time to prevent over-drying the skin.
5. Using a humidifier to add moisture to the air, particularly in dry or cold environments.
6. Considering prescription-strength moisturizers or keratolytic agents, such as topical retinoids or vitamin D analogs, to help manage more severe symptoms.

In some cases, individuals with ichthyosis vulgaris may also benefit from systemic treatments, such as oral retinoids, which can help to regulate skin cell turnover and improve skin texture. However, these treatments should only be used under the guidance of a qualified healthcare provider, as they can have significant side effects and risks.

10.3 Other Related Skin Conditions

In addition to atopic dermatitis and ichthyosis vulgaris, there are several other skin conditions that may be associated with Keratosis Pilaris or share similar features. These include:

1. Follicular eczema: Follicular eczema is a type of eczema that primarily affects the hair follicles, causing small, red, itchy bumps that may resemble KP. It is often triggered by exposure to irritants or allergens, and may be more common in individuals with a history of atopic dermatitis.

2. Pityriasis rubra pilaris: Pityriasis rubra pilaris (PRP) is a rare skin disorder characterized by red, scaly patches and follicular papules that may resemble KP. However, unlike KP, PRP often involves the palms, soles, and scalp, and may be associated with systemic symptoms like joint pain or fever.

3. Lichen spinulosus: Lichen spinulosus is a rare skin condition characterized by small, spiny papules that typically appear on the neck, trunk, and arms. While the exact cause is unknown, it is thought to be related to abnormal keratinization of the hair follicles, similar to KP.

4. Keratosis follicularis (Darier disease): Keratosis follicularis, also known as Darier disease, is a rare genetic disorder that causes wart-like papules and plaques to develop on the skin, particularly in areas of friction or sweating. While the lesions may resemble KP, they are typically larger and more pronounced, and may be associated with other symptoms like nail abnormalities or neuropsychiatric issues.

When managing KP in individuals with related skin conditions, it's important to work closely with a qualified dermatologist or healthcare provider to develop a personalized treatment plan that addresses the specific needs and concerns of each individual. This may involve a combination of topical or systemic treatments, lifestyle modifications, and preventive strategies to help manage symptoms and reduce the risk of flare-ups.

It's also important for individuals with KP and related skin conditions to be mindful of their overall health and well-being, as stress, poor nutrition, and other lifestyle factors can exacerbate symptoms and complicate treatment. Some strategies for supporting overall health and well-being may include:

1. Eating a balanced, nutrient-rich diet that includes plenty of fruits, vegetables, whole grains, and lean proteins.
2. Staying hydrated by drinking plenty of water and other fluids throughout the day.
3. Getting regular exercise and physical activity, which can help to reduce stress, improve circulation, and support healthy skin.
4. Practicing stress-reducing techniques like deep breathing, meditation, or yoga to help manage stress and promote relaxation.
5. Getting enough sleep each night to support healthy skin and overall well-being.
6. Avoiding triggers that exacerbate skin symptoms, such as harsh skincare products, hot showers, or tight clothing.

By taking a comprehensive, holistic approach to KP management that addresses both the specific skin concerns and the overall health and well-being of each individual, those with KP and related skin conditions can help to support healthy, comfortable skin and improve their quality of life.

In conclusion, while Keratosis Pilaris is a distinct skin condition, it is often associated with other skin disorders or systemic conditions that can complicate treatment and management. By understanding these associations and working closely with qualified healthcare providers, individuals with KP can develop personalized treatment plans that address their specific needs and concerns. Whether managing KP in the context of atopic dermatitis, ichthyosis vulgaris, or other related skin conditions, a comprehensive approach that includes gentle skincare, lifestyle modifications, and medical interventions as needed can help to support healthy, comfortable skin and improve overall quality of life. As with all aspects of KP management, patience, consistency, and self-compassion are key to achieving optimal results and maintaining long-term skin health.

CHAPTER 11

Makeup and Cosmetic Strategies for Keratosis Pilaris

Keratosis Pilaris (KP) can be a source of self-consciousness and insecurity for many individuals, particularly when the bumps and redness are visible on exposed areas of the skin. While makeup and cosmetic products cannot treat the underlying causes of KP, they can be valuable tools for concealing and minimizing the appearance of KP bumps and redness, helping individuals to feel more confident and comfortable in their skin. In this chapter, we'll explore some makeup and cosmetic strategies for managing the appearance of KP, from prepping the skin for makeup application to choosing the right products and techniques for a flawless finish.

11.1 Preparing the Skin for Makeup Application

Before applying any makeup or cosmetic products to KP-affected skin, it's important to properly prepare the skin to ensure a smooth, even application and minimize the risk of irritation or exacerbation of symptoms. Some key steps for prepping KP skin for makeup include:

1. Cleansing: Start by gently cleansing the skin with a mild, non-irritating cleanser that is appropriate for your skin type. Avoid harsh scrubs or exfoliants, which can irritate the skin and worsen KP bumps. Pat the skin dry with a soft, clean towel.

2. Moisturizing: Apply a lightweight, non-comedogenic moisturizer to help hydrate and soften the skin, creating a smooth base for makeup application. Look for moisturizers that contain ingredients like hyaluronic acid, glycerin, or dimethicone, which can help to plump and smooth the skin without clogging pores.

3. Priming: Consider using a makeup primer to help create an even, smooth canvas for foundation and concealer. Look for primers that are specifically formulated for textured or uneven skin, as these can help to fill in and smooth out KP bumps and rough patches. Silicone-based primers can be particularly effective for creating a smooth, even base.

4. Sunscreen: If you'll be spending time outdoors or exposing your skin to UV light, be sure to apply a broad-spectrum sunscreen with an SPF of at least 30 before applying makeup. Look for lightweight, non-greasy formulas that won't clog pores or exacerbate KP symptoms.

By taking the time to properly prep the skin before applying makeup, you can help to ensure a more even, natural-looking finish and minimize the risk of irritation or worsening of KP symptoms.

11.2 Choosing the Right Makeup Products

When it comes to choosing makeup products for KP-affected skin, it's important to look for formulas that are non-comedogenic, lightweight, and gentle on the skin. Some key products to consider include:

1. Color-correcting concealer: KP bumps and redness can be particularly challenging to conceal with traditional concealer alone. Using a color-correcting concealer in a green or yellow shade can help to neutralize redness and create a more even base for foundation. Look for creamy, blendable formulas that won't settle into or emphasize bumps or rough patches.

2. Lightweight foundation: When choosing a foundation for KP-affected skin, look for lightweight, non-comedogenic formulas that provide sheer to medium coverage. Avoid heavy, full-coverage foundations that can settle into and emphasize KP bumps. Consider using a damp beauty sponge or stippling brush to apply foundation, as these tools can help to create a more natural, skin-like finish.

3. Setting powder: To help set makeup and minimize the appearance of texture, consider using a lightweight, translucent setting powder. Look for finely milled powders that won't settle into or emphasize KP bumps, and apply with a fluffy brush or damp beauty sponge for a more natural finish.

4. Blush and bronzer: When applying blush and bronzer to KP-affected skin, look for sheer, buildable formulas that can be easily blended and diffused. Avoid heavy, pigmented formulas that can emphasize texture and unevenness. Consider using a fan brush or stippling brush to apply blush and bronzer, as these tools can help to create a more natural, diffused effect.

5. Highlighter: Highlighting products can be particularly challenging for KP-affected skin, as they can emphasize texture and unevenness. If you choose to use a highlighter, look for sheer, subtle formulas that can be easily blended and diffused. Consider using a small, fluffy brush to apply highlighter to the high points of the face, such as the cheekbones and brow bone, and blend well for a more natural effect.

When selecting makeup products for KP-affected skin, it's also important to choose formulas that are free from potential irritants or allergens, such as fragrances, dyes, or harsh preservatives. If you have sensitive or reactive skin, consider patch-testing new products before applying them to larger areas of the face or body.

11.3 Camouflage Techniques for Keratosis Pilaris

In addition to choosing the right makeup products, there are several techniques and strategies that can be effective for camouflaging and minimizing the appearance of KP bumps and redness. Some key techniques to consider include:

1. Color correction: As mentioned earlier, using a color-correcting concealer in a green or yellow shade can be an effective way to neutralize redness and create a more even base for foundation. To use a color-correcting concealer, apply a small amount of product directly to the areas of redness, and blend well with a small brush or fingertip. Follow with foundation and concealer as needed.

2. Stippling and blending: When applying foundation and concealer to KP-affected skin, it's important to use gentle, stippling motions rather than rubbing or dragging the product across the skin. This can help to minimize the appearance of texture and create a more natural, skin-like finish. Use a damp beauty sponge or stippling brush to gently press and blend the product into the skin, building up coverage as needed.

3. Layering: For more stubborn areas of redness or uneven texture, consider layering different types of products to achieve a more seamless finish. For example, you might start with a color-correcting concealer to neutralize redness, follow with a lightweight foundation to even out skin tone, and then spot-conceal any remaining bumps or imperfections with a high-coverage concealer.

4. Setting and finishing: To help set makeup and minimize the appearance of texture, be sure to use a lightweight setting powder or spray after applying foundation and concealer. Look for finely milled, translucent powders that won't settle into or emphasize bumps or rough patches. Use a fluffy brush or damp beauty sponge to gently press the powder into the skin, focusing on areas that tend to get oily or shiny throughout the day.

5. Blurring and diffusing: For a more airbrushed, perfected finish, consider using a blurring or diffusing product as a final step in your makeup routine. These products typically contain silicone or other skin-smoothing ingredients that can help to minimize the appearance of pores, fine lines, and uneven texture. Apply a small amount of product to the high points of the face, such as the cheekbones and forehead, and blend well with a brush or fingertips.

While these techniques can be effective for camouflaging and minimizing the appearance of KP bumps and redness, it's important to remember that they are not a substitute for proper skincare and treatment. Makeup and cosmetic products should be used in conjunction with a consistent skincare routine and any recommended medical treatments to achieve the best possible results.

It's also important to be gentle and patient when applying makeup to KP-affected skin, as aggressive rubbing or tugging can irritate the skin and worsen symptoms. Take your time, use gentle motions, and don't be afraid to experiment with different products and techniques until you find what works best for your individual skin type and concerns.

Finally, remember that while makeup and cosmetic products can be valuable tools for boosting confidence and self-esteem, they are not a requirement for beauty or self-worth. Embrace your unique skin and celebrate your natural beauty, with or without makeup. By practicing self-love and self-acceptance, you can develop a more positive and resilient relationship with your skin, regardless of the presence of KP or other imperfections.

In conclusion, makeup and cosmetic strategies can be valuable tools for individuals with Keratosis Pilaris who want to minimize the appearance of bumps and redness and feel more confident in their skin. By properly preparing the skin, choosing the right products, and using gentle, effective application techniques, it is possible to achieve a smooth, even, and natural-looking finish that can help to camouflage KP symptoms. However, it's important to remember that makeup is just one aspect of a comprehensive KP management plan, and should be used in conjunction with proper skincare, medical treatment, and self-care practices for optimal results. Ultimately, the goal of makeup and cosmetic strategies for KP should be to enhance and celebrate your unique beauty, not to hide or shame your natural skin. By approaching makeup with a spirit of self-love and self-acceptance, you can develop a more positive and empowered relationship with your skin, KP and all.

CHAPTER 12

Keratosis Pilaris and Self-Esteem: Embracing Your Skin

Keratosis Pilaris (KP) is a common skin condition that affects millions of people worldwide, but its impact extends far beyond the physical appearance of the skin. For many individuals with KP, the condition can take a significant toll on self-esteem and body image, leading to feelings of self-consciousness, embarrassment, and even shame. In this chapter, we'll explore the emotional impact of KP and discuss strategies for cultivating self-love, self-acceptance, and a more positive relationship with your skin.

12.1 Reframing Your Perspective on Keratosis Pilaris

One of the first steps in building a more positive relationship with your skin is to reframe your perspective on Keratosis Pilaris. It's easy to get caught up in negative self-talk and beliefs about KP, such as "my skin is ugly," "I'll never have smooth skin," or "people are judging me because of my KP." However, these thoughts are not only unhelpful, but they are also untrue.

KP is a common and medically harmless condition that affects people of all ages, races, and genders. It is not a reflection of your worth as a person, your hygiene, or your overall health. In fact, many people with KP go on to live happy, fulfilling lives and have successful relationships and careers, regardless of the appearance of their skin.

To start reframing your perspective on KP, try to catch yourself when you engage in negative self-talk or comparisons to others. Instead of focusing on what you perceive as flaws or imperfections, try to shift your attention to the unique qualities and strengths that make you who you are. Remember that your worth and value as a person are not determined by the texture or appearance of your skin.

It can also be helpful to educate yourself about KP and connect with others who share your experience. Learning more about the scientific causes and treatments for KP can help to demystify the condition and reduce feelings of shame or self-blame. Joining online support communities or attending in-person support groups can provide a sense of connection and validation, reminding you that you are not alone in your struggles with KP.

12.2 Practicing Self-Love and Acceptance

Building a more positive relationship with your skin also requires practicing self-love and acceptance on a daily basis. This means treating yourself with the same kindness, compassion, and respect that you would extend to a good friend or loved one.

One way to practice self-love is to engage in activities that make you feel good about yourself and your body, regardless of the appearance of your skin. This might include exercise, dance, yoga, or any other physical activity that helps you feel strong, capable, and connected to your body. It could also include creative pursuits like art, music, or writing, which allow you to express yourself and explore your unique talents and passions.

Another important aspect of self-love is self-care. This means taking the time to nurture and care for your physical, emotional, and mental health, even when you're feeling self-conscious or down about your skin. Some self-care practices that can be particularly helpful for individuals with KP include:

1. Developing a gentle, consistent skincare routine that focuses on hydration, moisture, and nourishment rather than harsh scrubbing or exfoliation.

2. Eating a balanced, nutrient-rich diet that supports overall health and well-being, rather than restricting or punishing yourself with strict diets or food rules.

3. Getting enough sleep and rest, which can help to reduce stress, support healthy skin function, and promote a more positive outlook on life.

4. Engaging in stress-reducing activities like deep breathing, meditation, or spending time in nature, which can help to calm the mind and promote a sense of inner peace and well-being.

5. Surrounding yourself with positive, supportive people who uplift and encourage you, rather than those who criticize or judge you based on your appearance.

Practicing self-acceptance means learning to embrace and appreciate your unique body and skin, even if it doesn't conform to societal standards of perfection. It means recognizing that your worth and value are inherent and unconditional, and not dependent on the approval or validation of others.

One way to cultivate self-acceptance is to practice gratitude for your body and all the amazing things it allows you to do, rather than focusing on perceived flaws or imperfections. Take a moment each day to appreciate the strength, resilience, and beauty of your body, and all the ways it supports you in living a fulfilling life.

Another helpful practice is to challenge and reframe negative thoughts and beliefs about your skin and appearance. When you catch yourself engaging in self-criticism or comparison, try to counter those thoughts with more realistic, compassionate ones. For example, instead of thinking "my skin is so ugly and embarrassing," try reframing it as "my skin is unique and beautiful in its own way, and does not define my worth as a person."

12.3 Inspiring Stories and Testimonials

One of the most powerful ways to cultivate self-love and acceptance is to seek out inspiring stories and testimonials from others who have learned to embrace their skin and live fulfilling lives with KP. Hearing about the experiences and triumphs of others can provide a sense of hope, validation, and connection, reminding you that you are not alone in your struggles and that it is possible to develop a more positive relationship with your skin.

There are many individuals with KP who have become advocates, role models, and voices of inspiration within the KP community. Some have shared their stories through social media, blogs, or videos, while others have written books, given interviews, or spoken publicly about their experiences. By seeking out and engaging with these stories, you can gain valuable insights, tips, and perspectives on living confidently and joyfully with KP.

For example, Nitika Chopra, a beauty and lifestyle expert who has lived with KP since childhood, has become a prominent voice in the KP community. Through her blog, social media presence, and public speaking engagements, she shares her journey of self-love and acceptance, and encourages others to embrace their unique beauty and worth, regardless of their skin condition.

Another inspiring figure is Jude Chao, a skincare blogger and advocate who has written extensively about her experiences with KP and other skin conditions. Through her blog, Fifty Shades of Snail, she provides practical tips, product recommendations, and emotional support for others struggling with KP and other skin concerns.

There are also many everyday individuals with KP who have shared their stories and experiences through online forums, support groups, and social media communities. By connecting with these individuals and hearing about their struggles and triumphs, you can gain a sense of perspective, inspiration, and solidarity in your own journey with KP.

Ultimately, the most inspiring story is your own. By committing to a journey of self-love, self-acceptance, and self-care, you can become your own role model and source of inspiration, not only for yourself but for others struggling with KP and similar skin conditions. Remember that your worth and value are inherent and unconditional, and that you have the power to create a more positive, fulfilling relationship with your skin and your body, one day at a time.

In conclusion, while Keratosis Pilaris can be a source of significant emotional distress and self-consciousness for many individuals, it is possible to cultivate a more positive, accepting relationship with your skin. By reframing your perspective on KP, practicing self-love and self-care, and seeking out inspiring stories and role models, you can learn to embrace your unique beauty and worth, regardless of the texture or appearance of your skin.

Remember that building self-esteem and body confidence is a journey, not a destination. There will be ups and downs, good days and bad days, but by committing to a practice of self-love and self-acceptance, you can develop greater resilience, compassion, and appreciation for yourself and your body.

It's also important to remember that you are not alone in your struggles with KP and self-esteem. There is a vast community of individuals who share your experiences and are here to support, encourage, and inspire you along the way. Don't hesitate to reach out for help, whether it's through online forums, support groups, or professional counseling services.

Ultimately, the goal is not to achieve perfect, flawless skin, but rather to develop a more peaceful, accepting relationship with the skin you have. By learning to love and appreciate yourself, KP and all, you can unlock a greater sense of confidence, joy, and fulfillment in all areas of your life. So embrace your unique beauty, celebrate your resilience, and know that you are worthy and valuable, just as you are.

CHAPTER 13

Preventing and Minimizing Keratosis Pilaris Flare-Ups

Keratosis Pilaris (KP) is a chronic skin condition that requires ongoing management and care to minimize the frequency and severity of flare-ups. While there is no cure for KP, there are several strategies and techniques that can help to prevent and reduce the occurrence of bumps, redness, and irritation associated with the condition. In this chapter, we'll explore some of the most effective ways to keep KP under control and maintain healthy, comfortable skin.

13.1 Identifying and Avoiding Triggers

One of the most important steps in preventing KP flare-ups is to identify and avoid potential triggers that can exacerbate symptoms. While the exact causes of KP are not fully understood, there are several factors that are known to contribute to the development and worsening of the condition. By becoming aware of these triggers and taking steps to minimize their impact, you can help to keep your KP under control and reduce the frequency and severity of flare-ups.

Some common triggers for KP include:

1. Dry skin: KP is often associated with dry, dehydrated skin, which can exacerbate the buildup of keratin and lead to the formation of rough, bumpy

patches. To keep your skin hydrated and minimize the risk of flare-ups, it's important to moisturize regularly with a rich, emollient cream or lotion, and to avoid harsh soaps, hot showers, and other drying agents.

2. Friction and irritation: Friction from tight clothing, rough fabrics, or aggressive scrubbing can irritate the skin and worsen KP symptoms. To minimize friction and irritation, opt for loose, breathable clothing made from soft, natural fibers like cotton or bamboo, and avoid harsh scrubs, loofahs, or other abrasive products.

3. Hormonal changes: Hormonal fluctuations, such as those that occur during puberty, pregnancy, or menopause, can trigger or worsen KP symptoms in some individuals. While it may not be possible to completely avoid these changes, being aware of their potential impact can help you to be more proactive in your skincare routine and take steps to minimize flare-ups.

4. Environmental factors: Exposure to cold, dry air, wind, or excessive sun can all contribute to the development and worsening of KP symptoms. To protect your skin from these environmental stressors, it's important to use a gentle, moisturizing sunscreen year-round, and to take steps to humidify your home or office during dry winter months.

5. Stress: Stress can have a significant impact on skin health, and can trigger or worsen KP symptoms in some individuals. To minimize the impact of stress on your skin, it's important to practice stress-reducing techniques like deep breathing, meditation, or yoga, and to prioritize self-care and relaxation in your daily routine.

By becoming aware of these potential triggers and taking steps to avoid or minimize their impact, you can help to prevent KP flare-ups and maintain healthier, more comfortable skin.

13.2 Maintaining a Consistent Skin Care Routine

Another key factor in preventing and minimizing KP flare-ups is maintaining a consistent, gentle skincare routine that focuses on hydration, exfoliation, and nourishment. While the specific products and techniques that work best may vary depending on your individual skin type and concerns, there are some general principles that can help to keep KP under control and promote overall skin health.

1. Cleanse gently: Avoid harsh, drying soaps or scrubs that can strip the skin of its natural oils and irritate KP-prone areas. Instead, opt for a gentle, fragrance-free cleanser that is designed for sensitive skin, and use lukewarm water to avoid over-drying or irritating the skin.

2. Exfoliate regularly: Regular exfoliation can help to prevent the buildup of keratin and dead skin cells that contribute to the formation of KP bumps. However, it's important to use gentle, non-abrasive exfoliants that won't irritate or damage the skin. Look for products that contain alpha-hydroxy acids (AHAs) like glycolic or lactic acid, or beta-hydroxy acids (BHAs) like salicylic acid, which can help to dissolve keratin plugs and promote cell turnover.

3. Moisturize deeply: Keeping the skin hydrated and nourished is essential for preventing and minimizing KP flare-ups. Look for rich, emollient moisturizers that contain ingredients like urea, ceramides, or hyaluronic acid, which can help to attract and retain moisture in the skin. Apply moisturizer immediately after bathing or showering to lock in hydration, and reapply throughout the day as needed.

4. Protect from the sun: Sun exposure can dry out and irritate KP-prone skin, leading to increased redness, inflammation, and flare-ups. To protect your skin from the sun's harmful rays, use a gentle, moisturizing sunscreen with an SPF of at least 30 every day, even on cloudy or overcast days. Look for products that are specifically designed for sensitive or irritation-prone skin, and reapply every 2 hours or after swimming or sweating.

5. Be patient and consistent: Building and maintaining a healthy skincare routine takes time and consistency. Don't expect overnight results, and don't get discouraged if you experience occasional flare-ups or setbacks. Stick with your routine, make adjustments as needed based on your skin's response, and be patient with the process. Over time, a consistent, gentle skincare routine can help to improve the overall health and appearance of your skin and minimize the impact of KP.

In addition to these basic principles, there are some specific products and ingredients that may be particularly helpful for managing KP and preventing flare-ups. These include:

- Topical retinoids: Retinoids like tretinoin or adapalene can help to regulate cell turnover and reduce the buildup of keratin in the hair follicles. However, these products can be drying and irritating for some individuals, so it's important to start with a low concentration and gradually increase as tolerated, under the guidance of a dermatologist.

- Chemical exfoliants: As mentioned earlier, AHAs and BHAs can be effective for gently exfoliating the skin and reducing the appearance of KP bumps. Look for products that contain glycolic, lactic, or salicylic acid in concentrations of 5-10%, and use 1-2 times per week as tolerated.

- Prescription-strength moisturizers: For more severe or stubborn cases of KP, your dermatologist may recommend a prescription-strength moisturizer that contains higher concentrations of ingredients like urea, lactic acid, or ceramides. These products can provide more intensive hydration and exfoliation to help manage KP symptoms.

By developing and maintaining a consistent, gentle skincare routine that focuses on hydration, exfoliation, and sun protection, you can help to prevent and minimize KP flare-ups and promote overall skin health and comfort.

13.3 Strategies for Long-Term Management

While a consistent skincare routine and avoidance of triggers can go a long way in managing KP symptoms, there are also some long-term strategies and lifestyle factors that can help to keep the condition under control and promote overall skin health. These include:

1. Eating a healthy, balanced diet: While there is no specific diet that has been proven to cure or prevent KP, eating a balanced, nutrient-rich diet can help to support overall skin health and minimize inflammation in the body. Focus on whole, unprocessed foods like fruits, vegetables, whole grains, and lean proteins, and limit your intake of sugar, refined carbohydrates, and unhealthy fats.

2. Staying hydrated: Drinking plenty of water throughout the day can help to keep your skin hydrated from the inside out, which can minimize the appearance of dry, flaky patches and reduce the risk of KP flare-ups. Aim for at least 8 glasses of water per day, and more if you are physically active or live in a dry climate.

3. Managing stress: Stress can have a significant impact on skin health, and can trigger or worsen KP symptoms in some individuals. To minimize the impact of stress on your skin, it's important to develop healthy coping mechanisms and stress-reducing practices, such as deep breathing, meditation, exercise, or spending time in nature.

4. Avoiding harsh or irritating products: Many skincare and household products contain harsh chemicals, fragrances, or other irritants that can exacerbate KP symptoms and damage the skin's natural barrier function. To minimize irritation and sensitivity, opt for gentle, fragrance-free products that are specifically designed for sensitive skin, and avoid harsh scrubs, exfoliants, or other abrasive products.

5. Treating underlying health conditions: In some cases, KP may be associated with underlying health conditions such as atopic dermatitis, thyroid disorders, or vitamin deficiencies. If you suspect that your KP may be related to an underlying health issue, it's important to speak with your healthcare provider and receive appropriate testing and treatment. Addressing these underlying conditions can often help to improve KP symptoms and overall skin health.

6. Considering professional treatments: For more severe or stubborn cases of KP, professional treatments such as chemical peels, microdermabrasion, or laser therapy may be recommended by your dermatologist. These treatments can help to exfoliate the skin, reduce the appearance of bumps and redness, and promote cell turnover for smoother, clearer skin.

7. Being patient and persistent: Managing KP is a long-term process that requires patience, consistency, and a willingness to experiment with different strategies and products to find what works best for your individual skin type and concerns. Don't get discouraged if you experience setbacks or flare-ups along the way – with time and persistence, it is possible to achieve significant improvements in the appearance and comfort of your skin.

By incorporating these long-term management strategies into your overall skincare routine and lifestyle, you can help to prevent and minimize KP flare-ups, promote overall skin health, and feel more confident and comfortable in your own skin.

In conclusion, preventing and minimizing Keratosis Pilaris flare-ups requires a multi-faceted approach that includes identifying and avoiding triggers, maintaining a consistent skincare routine, and adopting long-term management strategies that support overall skin health and well-being. While there is no one-size-fits-all solution for managing KP, by experimenting with different products, techniques, and lifestyle factors, it is possible to find a combination that works best for your individual needs and concerns.

Remember, managing KP is a journey, not a destination. There will be ups and downs, good days and bad days, but by staying committed to your skincare routine and overall health, you can achieve significant improvements in the appearance and comfort of your skin over time. Don't hesitate to seek support and guidance from a dermatologist or other skincare professional if you need help developing a personalized treatment plan or managing more severe or stubborn symptoms.

Most importantly, be kind and patient with yourself throughout the process. Your worth and value are not determined by the appearance of your skin, and it's important to practice self-love and self-acceptance even as you work towards your skincare goals. Celebrate your unique beauty and resilience, and remember that you are so much more than your KP. With time, consistency, and a positive outlook, you can learn to manage your KP with confidence and grace, and live your best life with healthy, comfortable skin.

CHAPTER 14

The Future of Keratosis Pilaris Treatment: Research and Innovations

Keratosis Pilaris (KP) is a common skin condition that affects millions of people worldwide, yet there is still much to be learned about its underlying causes, risk factors, and most effective treatment options. While current treatments can help to manage symptoms and improve the appearance of KP-affected skin, there is no cure for the condition, and many individuals continue to struggle with persistent bumps, redness, and irritation. However, ongoing research and innovations in the field of dermatology offer hope for the future of KP treatment, with the potential for more targeted, effective, and long-lasting solutions.

14.1 Current Research and Clinical Trials

One area of active research in the field of KP treatment is the investigation of new and emerging therapies that target the underlying causes of the condition. While the exact pathophysiology of KP is not fully understood, it is thought to involve a combination of genetic, environmental, and immunological factors that lead to the overproduction and buildup of keratin in the hair follicles. By better understanding these underlying mechanisms, researchers hope to develop more precise and effective treatments that can address the root causes of KP and provide longer-lasting relief.

Some of the current research and clinical trials related to KP treatment include:

1. Topical retinoids: Retinoids are a class of compounds derived from vitamin A that have been shown to regulate cell turnover, reduce inflammation, and improve the appearance of KP-affected skin. While topical retinoids like tretinoin and adapalene are already used in the treatment of KP, ongoing research is investigating new formulations and delivery methods that may enhance their efficacy and tolerability.

2. Laser and light therapies: Laser and light-based treatments have shown promise in the management of KP, with the ability to target and reduce the appearance of red, inflamed bumps and promote collagen production for smoother, clearer skin. Current research is exploring the use of new laser technologies, such as fractional lasers and intense pulsed light (IPL), as well as optimizing treatment protocols for maximum safety and efficacy.

3. Microneedling: Microneedling is a minimally invasive procedure that involves the use of fine needles to create micro-injuries in the skin, stimulating collagen production and promoting cell turnover. While microneedling has been used in the treatment of various skin conditions, including acne scars and hyperpigmentation, recent studies have suggested that it may also be effective in reducing the appearance of KP bumps and improving overall skin texture.

4. Biologic therapies: Biologic therapies are a newer class of medications that target specific immune system pathways involved in the development of inflammatory skin conditions. While biologics have primarily been used in the treatment of psoriasis and atopic dermatitis, ongoing research is investigating their potential use in the management of KP, particularly in cases that are resistant to traditional therapies.

5. Nutritional interventions: While the role of diet in the development and management of KP is not fully understood, some studies have suggested that

certain nutritional factors, such as vitamin A and omega-3 fatty acids, may play a role in skin health and the severity of KP symptoms. Ongoing research is exploring the potential benefits of dietary modifications and nutritional supplements in the management of KP, as well as their optimal dosing and formulation.

These are just a few examples of the current research and clinical trials related to KP treatment, and there arc likely many more exciting developments on the horizon. As our understanding of the underlying causes and mechanisms of KP continues to grow, so too will our ability to develop more targeted, effective, and personalized treatment options for those affected by this common skin condition.

14.2 Promising New Treatments on the Horizon

In addition to the ongoing research and clinical trials, there are several promising new treatments for KP that are currently in development or have recently become available. These innovative therapies offer the potential for more effective, convenient, and long-lasting management of KP symptoms, and may represent significant advances in the field of dermatology.

Some of the most promising new treatments for KP include:

1. Topical probiotics: Probiotics are beneficial bacteria that have been shown to play a role in skin health by modulating the immune system and promoting a healthy skin microbiome. Recent studies have suggested that topical probiotics, such as those containing specific strains of Lactobacillus or Bifidobacterium, may be effective in reducing inflammation and improving the appearance of KP-affected skin. While more research is needed to fully understand the potential benefits and optimal formulation of topical probiotics for KP, this emerging therapy offers a promising new approach to managing the condition.

2. Nanoparticle-based drug delivery: Nanoparticle-based drug delivery systems are a cutting-edge technology that allows for the targeted delivery of therapeutic compounds to specific cells or tissues in the body. In the context of KP treatment, nanoparticle-based systems could potentially allow for the precise delivery of keratolytic agents, retinoids, or other active ingredients directly to the affected hair follicles, minimizing systemic absorption and reducing the risk of side effects. While still in the early stages of development, nanoparticle-based therapies offer an exciting new frontier in the treatment of KP and other skin conditions.

3. Combination therapies: While many current KP treatments focus on a single active ingredient or mechanism of action, emerging research suggests that combination therapies, which use multiple active ingredients with complementary effects, may be more effective in managing the condition. For example, a combination of a topical retinoid with a keratolytic agent like urea or lactic acid may provide synergistic benefits in terms of reducing keratin buildup, promoting cell turnover, and improving skin hydration. As our understanding of the complex interplay between different therapeutic agents grows, we may see more advanced combination therapies become available for the treatment of KP.

4. Personalized medicine: One of the most promising areas of innovation in the field of dermatology is the development of personalized medicine, which involves tailoring treatment approaches to the unique genetic, environmental, and lifestyle factors of each individual patient. In the context of KP, this could involve the use of genetic testing to identify specific mutations or risk factors that may influence the severity or treatment response of the condition, as well as the development of customized treatment plans that take into account factors like skin type, age, and overall health status. While still in its early stages, personalized medicine offers the potential for more precise, effective, and well-tolerated treatments for KP and other skin conditions.

As these and other promising new treatments continue to be developed and refined, it is likely that we will see significant advances in the management of KP in the coming years. However, it is important to note that the development of new therapies is a complex and time-consuming process, and it may be several years before some of these innovative approaches become widely available to patients. In the meantime, individuals with KP can work closely with their dermatologists to develop personalized treatment plans that incorporate the best available evidence-based therapies, along with healthy lifestyle practices and self-care strategies.

14.3 Advocating for Keratosis Pilaris Awareness and Research Funding

While ongoing research and innovations offer hope for the future of KP treatment, it is important to recognize that progress in this area is often limited by a lack of awareness and funding for the condition. Despite affecting millions of people worldwide, KP is often considered a cosmetic concern rather than a medical condition, and as a result, it may not receive the same level of attention or resources as other skin disorders.

To help accelerate the pace of research and innovation in KP treatment, it is essential for individuals affected by the condition, as well as their families, friends, and healthcare providers, to become advocates for increased awareness and funding. Some ways to get involved and make a difference include:

1. Educating others: One of the most important ways to raise awareness about KP is to educate others about the condition, its impact on quality of life, and the need for more effective treatments. This can involve sharing personal stories and experiences, as well as promoting accurate and up-to-date information about KP through social media, blogs, or other online platforms.

2. Supporting advocacy organizations: There are several organizations and foundations dedicated to advancing research and awareness of skin

conditions, including the National Keratosis Pilaris Association (NKPA) and the American Academy of Dermatology (AAD). By supporting these organizations through donations, volunteering, or participating in events and campaigns, individuals can help to raise the profile of KP and advocate for increased funding and resources.

3. Participating in research studies: One of the most direct ways to contribute to the advancement of KP treatment is to participate in research studies and clinical trials. By volunteering to take part in these studies, individuals can help researchers to better understand the underlying causes and potential treatments for KP, as well as provide valuable data on the safety and efficacy of new therapies.

4. Advocating for policy change: Another important way to support KP research and awareness is to advocate for policy changes at the local, state, and national levels. This can involve contacting elected officials to express support for increased funding for dermatological research, as well as advocating for policies that improve access to healthcare and insurance coverage for individuals with KP and other skin conditions.

5. Building a supportive community: Finally, one of the most valuable ways to promote KP awareness and research is to build a supportive community of individuals affected by the condition. By connecting with others who share similar experiences and challenges, individuals can find validation, encouragement, and practical advice for managing KP, as well as work together to raise awareness and advocate for change.

As more individuals and organizations become involved in advocating for KP awareness and research funding, it is likely that we will see accelerated progress in the development of new and more effective treatments for this common and often underappreciated skin condition. By working together and staying committed to the cause, we can help to improve the lives of millions of people affected by KP and bring us closer to a future where this condition is better understood, more effectively treated, and ultimately, cured.

In conclusion, the future of Keratosis Pilaris treatment is bright, with ongoing research and innovations offering the potential for more targeted, effective, and long-lasting solutions for this common skin condition. From topical probiotics and nanoparticle-based drug delivery systems to personalized medicine and combination therapies, there are many exciting developments on the horizon that could revolutionize the way we approach KP management.

However, realizing the full potential of these advances will require a concerted effort from individuals, organizations, and policymakers to raise awareness about KP, advocate for increased research funding, and support the development and accessibility of new treatments. By becoming informed, engaged, and empowered advocates for the KP community, we can help to accelerate progress and bring hope to the millions of people affected by this condition worldwide.

As we look to the future, it is important to remain optimistic and committed to the cause, while also being patient and realistic about the challenges and timelines involved in bringing new treatments to market. In the meantime, individuals with KP can work closely with their dermatologists to develop personalized management plans that incorporate the best available therapies, lifestyle practices, and self-care strategies, while also staying informed about the latest research and innovations in the field.

Ultimately, by working together and staying focused on the goal of improving the lives of those affected by KP, we can help to build a future where this condition is better understood, more effectively treated, and ultimately, overcome. So let us continue to advocate, educate, and innovate, and look forward to a brighter, clearer, and more comfortable future for all those living with Keratosis Pilaris.

CONCLUSION

Throughout this comprehensive guide, we have explored the many facets of Keratosis Pilaris, from its underlying causes and risk factors to the latest advances in treatment and management. We have seen how this common skin condition, characterized by its rough, bumpy texture and reddish appearance, can have a profound impact on the lives of those affected, both physically and emotionally. Yet, we have also discovered that with the right combination of knowledge, support, and personalized care, it is possible to effectively manage KP and achieve clearer, smoother, and more comfortable skin.

At the heart of this journey is a commitment to self-education and empowerment. By taking the time to understand the complex interplay of genetic, environmental, and immunological factors that contribute to KP, as well as the various treatment options and lifestyle strategies available, individuals can become active participants in their own care and advocate for their unique needs and goals. This may involve working closely with a dermatologist to develop a customized management plan, experimenting with different skincare products and routines to find what works best for their individual skin type and concerns, and making healthy lifestyle choices that support overall skin health and well-being.

Of course, managing Keratosis Pilaris is not always a straightforward or easy process. As we have seen, the condition can be stubborn, unpredictable, and at times, frustrating, with flare-ups and setbacks that can test even the most dedicated and optimistic of individuals. However, it is in these moments of challenge that the true power of knowledge, support, and resilience shines through. By staying informed about the latest research and treatment options, connecting with others who understand and share their experiences, and maintaining a positive and persistent attitude, individuals with KP can weather the ups and downs of their journey and emerge stronger, more confident, and more in control of their skin health.

Looking to the future, there is much reason for hope and excitement in the world of Keratosis Pilaris treatment and research. With ongoing advances in fields like topical probiotics, nanoparticle-based drug delivery, and personalized medicine, we are on the cusp of a new era of more targeted, effective, and long-lasting solutions for this common skin condition. As our understanding of the underlying mechanisms and risk factors of KP continues to grow, so too will our ability to develop novel therapies and management strategies that can help to minimize symptoms, prevent flare-ups, and ultimately, improve quality of life for those affected.

However, realizing the full potential of these advances will require more than just scientific progress. It will also require a concerted effort from individuals, organizations, and policymakers to raise awareness about KP, advocate for increased research funding and accessibility of care, and support the development and implementation of new treatments and management approaches. By becoming informed, engaged, and empowered advocates for the KP community, we can help to accelerate the pace of progress and ensure that the benefits of these innovations are felt by all those who need them most.

This is where the power of personal stories and experiences comes in. Throughout this book, we have heard from individuals who have faced the challenges of KP with courage, resilience, and grace, and who have found ways to thrive and flourish despite the obstacles in their path. These stories serve as a reminder that while KP may be a common thread that brings us together, it is our unique journeys, perspectives, and triumphs that define who we are and what we can achieve. By sharing our experiences and insights with others, we can help to build a stronger, more connected, and more empowered community of individuals living with KP, and inspire future generations to continue the fight for better treatments, greater awareness, and ultimately, a cure.

As we conclude this exploration of Keratosis Pilaris, it is important to remember that this is not the end of the journey, but rather the beginning of a new chapter. Armed with the knowledge, strategies, and support outlined in this guide, individuals with KP can face the future with confidence, knowing that they have the tools and resources they need to effectively manage their condition and live their best lives. Whether you are newly diagnosed or have been living with KP for years, know that you are not alone, and that there is always hope for clearer, smoother, and more comfortable skin on the horizon.

So let us move forward together, united in our commitment to education, advocacy, and innovation, and in our belief that every individual deserves to feel confident, comfortable, and in control of their skin health. Let us continue to share our stories, support one another, and push for progress, knowing that with each step, we are bringing ourselves closer to a future where Keratosis Pilaris is not just manageable, but fully understood and effectively treated.

To all those living with KP, remember that your worth and value extend far beyond the appearance of your skin. You are strong, resilient, and uniquely beautiful, and your journey with this condition is just one part of the rich tapestry of your life. Embrace your experiences, celebrate your triumphs, and never lose sight of the power and potential that lies within you.

The future of Keratosis Pilaris treatment is bright, and together, we can help to shape it into a reality that brings hope, healing, and empowerment to all those affected. So let us move forward with courage, compassion, and a steadfast commitment to the belief that clear, smooth, and comfortable skin is not just a possibility, but a promise. The journey may be long and the path may be winding, but with the right knowledge, support, and determination, there is nothing we cannot achieve.

* 9 7 9 8 3 3 4 1 2 0 0 0 6 *